Diagnosis and Man
Renal and Urinary

CW00371550

J. MICHAEL BOULTON JONES
MA MB BChir MRCP
Consultant Physician and Nephrologist
Royal Infirmary, Glasgow

J. DOUGLAS BRIGGS
MB ChB FRCPG
Consultant Nephrologist
Western Infirmary, Glasgow

TIMOTHY B. HARGREAVE
MB BS FRCS
Honorary Consultant Urologist and Transplant Surgeon
Western General Hospital, Edinburgh
Senior Lecturer in Surgical Urology
University of Edinburgh

BLACKWELL SCIENTIFIC PUBLICATIONS
OXFORD LONDON EDINBURGH
BOSTON MELBOURNE

© 1982 by
Blackwell Scientific Publications
Editorial offices:
Osney Mead, Oxford, OX2 0EL
8 John Street, London, WC1N 2ES
9 Forrest Road, Edinburgh, EH1 2QH
52 Beacon Street, Boston
   Massachusetts 02108, USA
99 Barry Street, Carlton,
   Victoria 3053, Australia

First published 1982

Typeset by
Scottish Studios & Engravers Ltd,
Glasgow
Printed and bound in Great Britain by
The Pitman Press, Bath

DISTRIBUTORS

USA
   Blackwell Mosby Book
   Distributors,
   11830 Westline Industrial Drive,
   St. Louis, Missouri 63141

Canada
   Blackwell Mosby Book
   Distributors,
   120 Melford Drive, Scarborough,
   Ontario, M1B 2X4

Australia
   Blackwell Scientific Book
   Distributors,
   214 Berkeley Street, Carlton,
   Victoria 3053

British Library
Cataloguing in Publication Data

Boulton Jones, J. Michael
   Diagnosis and management of renal
   and urinary diseases.
   1. Kidneys—Diseases
   2. Urinary organs—Diseases
   I. Title   II. Briggs, J. Douglas
   III. Hargreave, Timothy B.
   616.6'1   RC902

   ISBN 0632–00677–3

1529

iv

Contents

Preface

This book sets out the clinical problems posed by patients with disorders of the kidneys and urinary tract and describes their management. It inevitably reflects to a certain extent the personal views and beliefs of the authors. Renal diseases (apart from infections) .are uncommon; it is hoped that this book will help clinicians working in and out of hospitals to make their decisions with greater confidence and speed. The purpose is not to describe theoretical and experimental aspects of nephrology and urology. However, the book contains enough information to enable any student to face the MRCP examiners glowing with confidence, at least as far as the renal tract is concerned.

JMBJ
JDB
TBH November 1981

Anatomy and physiology of the kidney

ANATOMY

Gross anatomy

The kidneys lie behind the peritoneum on either side of the vertebral column. In the adult, each kidney measures around 13 to 15 cm in its long axis and together they weigh about 300 grams, that is about 0·4 per cent of the body weight. The gross anatomy of the kidney is illustrated in Figure 1.1. The outer surface is covered by a tough capsule beneath which lies the cortex. The deeper part of the cortex, the renal columns, lie between the pyramids which form the chief components of the medulla. The pyramids show fan-like striations due to the loops of Henle and blood vessels running in parallel. The innermost portion of each pyramid is the papilla, at the tip of which the ducts of Bellini discharge into the minor calyces. These in turn lead into the major calyces and the pelvis. The space within which the pelvis and calyces lie is the renal sinus and this also holds blood vessels and fat. The major blood vessels, ureter, lymphatics and nerves enter or leave the sinus at the hilum which occupies the middle third of the medial border of the kidney.

Nephron

These individual units, of which there are one to one and a quarter million in each kidney, are composed of the renal corpuscle (glomerulus and Bowman's capsule), proximal convoluted tubule, loop of Henle and distal convoluted tubule (Fig. 1.2). Many nephrons drain into each collecting duct and these in turn join to form the ducts of Bellini. Two types of nephrons can be

1

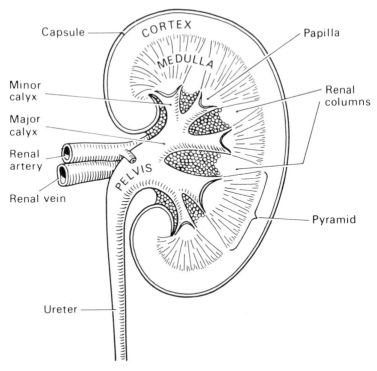

FIG. 1.1   Longitudinal section showing the main features of the kidney.

distinguished depending on their site. The cortical nephrons lie in the outer two-thirds of the cortex and have short loops of Henle which reach to, or just beyond, the cortico-medullary junction. The juxtamedullary nephrons lie in the inner third of the cortex and have long thin loops which extend deep into the medulla. To give some idea of the total length of tubules, if all nephrons from both kidneys were laid end to end they would stretch for 75 miles.

Vascular anatomy

Usually each kidney is supplied by one artery although the presence of two or more is fairly common. The artery divides into the interlobar branches which run between the pyramids to the cortico-medullary junction (Fig. 1.3). There they turn to run along this

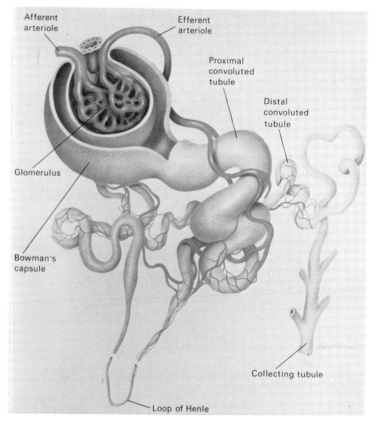

FIG. 1.2 The nephron showing the distal tubule returning to lie in apposition to the glomerulus from which it arose. The major part of the descending and ascending thin limbs of Henle's loop are not shown in the diagram. Reproduced with the permission of Smith, Kline & French Laboratories Ltd.

junction in a series of arches as the arcuate arteries. From there, the interlobular arteries arise at right angles and run through the cortex to the capsule, giving off the afferent arterioles, each of which runs to a glomerulus. As the afferent arteriole enters Bowman's capsule it is closely related to a segment of the distal tubule to form the juxtaglomerular apparatus. This is the site of renin secretion and consists of the specially modified cells of the arteriole (polkissen) which contain renin granules, the distal tubular cells (macula densa)

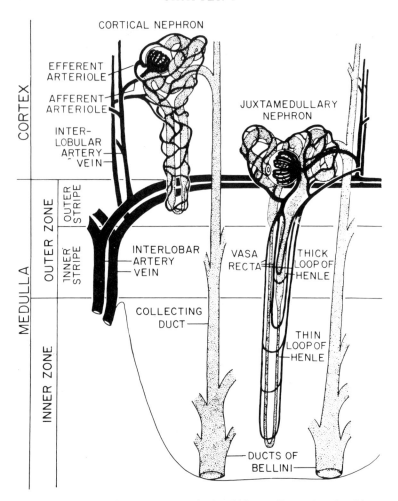

FIG. 1.3 Vascular anatomy of the kidney. Reproduced with permission from Pitts, R. F. (1974) *Physiology of the Kidney and Body Fluids*, Chicago: Year Book.

and in between a third type, the lacis cells (Fig. 1.4). The glomerulus consists of some 20–40 capillary loops and these lead into the efferent arteriole. From the cortical nephron, this in turn leads to the capillary network around the proximal and distal tubules. However, a more complex system pertains to the juxtamedullary nephron in that the efferent arteriole also gives rise

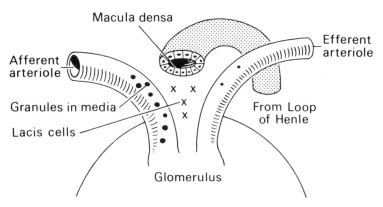

FIG. 1.4 Juxtaglomerular apparatus, consisting of the modified cells of the afferent arteriole (polkissen), the cells of the distal tubule (macula densa) and, in between, the lacis cells.

to long capillary loops, the vasa recta, which accompany the loop of Henle deep into the medulla, so enabling the countercurrent multiplier system to operate (see p. 14).

Glomerular ultrastructure

There are three layers between the glomerular capillary lumen and Bowman's space; the endothelial and epithelial cell cytoplasm and the basement membrane in between. Electron microscopy (Fig. 1.5) has shown that the endothelial cytoplasm has rounded, punched-out areas called fenestrations, while the epithelial layer consists of interdigitating foot processes or pedicels, the spaces between them being known as slit pores.

Tubular histology

The epithelial cells lining the tubular lumen vary markedly as one moves down the tubule. The proximal tubule is lined by cuboidal cells with basal nuclei, coarsely granular cytoplasm, and numerous cytoplasmic filaments lining the lumen. The initial convoluted portion leads on to a straight part, the descending thick limb of Henle's loop. This gives way to the descending and then ascending thin limbs of the loop of Henle, lined by flattened cells. The final portion is the distal tubule. As with the proximal tubule, there is a

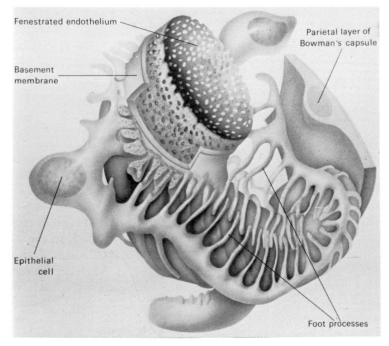

Fenestrated endothelium

Parietal layer of
Bowman's capsule

Basement
membrane

Epithelial
cell

Foot processes

FIG. 1.5   Diagrammatic representation of the three layers of the
glomerular capillary wall, the endothelium, basement membrane and
the epithelial cells with their foot processes. Reproduced with the
permission of Smith, Kline & French Laboratories Ltd.

straight length, the ascending thick limb of Henle's loop and a
convoluted part. The straight part is lined by cuboidal cells and the
convoluted part by columnar cells. The distal tubule in turn leads
into the collecting duct.

PHYSIOLOGY

Renal blood flow

The substance initially used to measure renal plasma flow (RPF) in
man was para amino hippurate (PAH), utilising the Fick principle:

$$RPF = \frac{\text{Urine conc. of PAH} \times \text{Urine volume}}{\text{Renal artery conc. of PAH} - \text{Renal vein conc. of PAH}}$$

As PAH clearance is 90 per cent complete in one passage through the kidney, and PAH is not extracted by other organs, the measurement is much simplified to:

$$RPF = \frac{\text{Urine conc. of PAH} \times \text{Urine volume}}{\text{Peripheral vein conc. of PAH}}$$

Thus PAH clearance is equal to about 90 per cent of total RPF. As PAH is extracted by the renal tubules, it is important to appreciate that it will not accurately measure RPF in the presence of tubular damage, i.e. in the diseased kidney. The use of Hippuran labelled with radioactive iodine, e.g. [131] I, provides a much simpler method of measuring RPF than PAH as the radioactivity in the samples can be rapidly counted rather than using chemical measurement. Also a single injection method has been developed which requires only serial plasma samples and no urine collection. However, Hippuran is only 80–85 per cent extracted in one passage through the kidney and correction of the result is needed to give the true RPF. The average RPF in the adult as measured by PAH clearance is 660 ml per minute.

Assuming a haematocrit of 45 per cent, renal blood flow (RBF) is:

$$RPF \times \left(\frac{1}{1 - \text{haematocrit}}\right) = 1200 \text{ ml per minute}$$

The cardiac output at rest is five to six litres per minute, and therefore just under 25 per cent of it supplies the kidneys. Accurate measurement of the distribution of blood flow within the human kidney is difficult but animal experiments suggest that 90 per cent goes to the cortex, 8–10 per cent to the medulla and 1–2 per cent to the papillae.

The control of RBF is by an extrinsic and an intrinsic system.

Extrinsic control. Various stimuli such as fear, pain, cold, exercise and haemorrhage lead to a reduction in RBF. It is difficult to be certain of the mechanism involved in each case but the two main pathways are the sympathetic nerves to the kidney which, of course, are vasoconstrictor, and hormones. The most important hormones, also vasoconstrictor, are adrenaline, noradrenaline and angiotensin II.

Intrinsic control. The maintenance of a stable RBF in the face of varying arterial pressure is essential to maintain a steady glomerular filtration rate (GFR). It is clear that this autoregulation of RBF occurs under the influence of intrinsic control mechanisms, although the precise nature of these mechanisms remains speculative.

RENIN-ANGIOTENSIN SYSTEM

The enzyme renin which is secreted by the juxtaglomerular apparatus acts on angiotensinogen to produce angiotensin I. This in turn is acted on by a converting enzyme to produce angiotensin II. This hormone is a potent vasoconstrictor and its most clearcut effect is to raise blood pressure. It is also one of the mediators of aldosterone secretion so indirectly has a sodium-retaining effect. Two trigger mechanisms are thought to control renin release. The first is a reduction in afferent arteriolar pressure which stimulates the polkissen. The other is an increase in the concentration of sodium in the tubular fluid reaching the macula densa. In addition to its role in the extrinsic control of RBF, the renin-angiotensin system is thought to play a part in the intrinsic control system. Its role presumably is to increase arteriolar tone in the presence of a reduction in renal blood flow.

Glomerular filtration

The passage of fluid and solutes through the glomerular capillary wall does not involve the expenditure of energy. Rather it consists of filtration, the most important determinant being molecular size. Up to a molecular weight of 5000 there is complete filtration, i.e. the concentration in the glomerular filtrate is the same as in the plasma. Thereafter the clearance falls progressively to virtually zero at a molecular weight of about 80000, i.e. around the molecular weight of albumin. In addition to molecular size, filtration is influenced by other factors. On the one hand is the hydrostatic pressure within the capillaries and opposing this are such forces as viscous drag and electrical and steric hindrance. Of these opposing forces, the electrical charge is probably the one of most importance. Positively charged molecules are more easily filtered than negatively charged ones of the same molecular size. This is because the glomerular basement membrane and the foot processes of the epithelial cells are covered by negatively charged molecules which repel others of a similar charge, thus reducing their rate of filtration. This surface negative charge appears to be lost in most glomerular diseases and is a major factor in the pathophysiology of proteinuria.

Calculation of glomerular filtration rate (GFR) requires measurement of the renal clearance of a substance which is freely filtered by the glomeruli and neither reabsorbed nor secreted by the tubules. Other criteria of the ideal substance are that it should be easily measured and not metabolized in the body. The renal clearance is defined as the number of millilitres of plasma completely cleared of the substance in one minute and the formula used is:

$$GFR = \frac{\text{Urine conc.} \times \text{Urine volume (ml per min)}}{\text{Plasma conc.}}$$

Inulin clearance accurately reflects GFR as inulin meets all these criteria except that its chemical measurement is tedious. More recently [131]I Hypaque and ^{51}Cr EDTA have been used. These too are accurate and have the important advantage of the ease of radioactive counting. In addition, as with the use of [131]I Hippuran to measure RPF, a single injection technique has been developed which requires only serial blood samples and no urine collections. Although less accurate, the endogenous creatinine clearance is still the most widely used method as it avoids the need for administration of any foreign substance, and the biochemical measurement of creatinine is routinely available. Secretion of creatinine by the renal tubules gives a result slightly above the true GFR but one which is accurate enough for most routine clinical purposes. GFR measurements should be adjusted to take account of varying body size and this is done by correcting the result to the standard body surface area of 1.73 m^2. The patient's surface area can be obtained from height and weight tables. When related to surface area there is a rise of GFR during the first two years of life, then the figure remains constant till around 60 years, followed by a slow decline. The normal values are 125 ± 15 ml per min per 1.73 m^2

surface area in males and 110 ± 15 ml per min per $1\cdot73$ m^2 surface area in females.

Tubular reabsorption

Massive quantities of water and solutes are reabsorbed through the tubular epithelial cells. Reabsorption can be either active or passive and active reabsorption can be by mechanisms exhibiting transport maxima (Tm) or gradient time limitation of transport capacity.

TM LIMITED MECHANISM

This type is characterised by a maximum capacity (Tm) of the tubules to reabsorb the substance which can be expressed in milligrams or millimoles per minute. If the quantity presented to the tubules exceeds the Tm, the excess will appear in the urine. Substances reabsorbed in this way include glucose, phosphate, sulphate, some amino acids and albumin. For example, although the concentration of albumin in the glomerular filtrate is very low at about 200 mg/l, this amounts to 32 g/24 hours. The Tm for albumin is about 30 mg/min, equivalent to 43 g/24 hours. Thus under normal circumstances the Tm is not exceeded and the urine is virtually albumin free. However, increased glomerular leakage of protein will rapidly overwhelm the reabsorptive capacity leading to proteinuria. All Tm limited reabsorption takes place in the proximal tubule.

GRADIENT TIME LIMITED MECHANISM

This mechanism controls sodium reabsorption in the proximal tubule, and is the main energy consuming function of the kidney, accounting for six per cent of the resting metabolism of man. As the name implies, reabsorption is related to the sodium gradient established across the tubular wall and the time the fluid is in contact with the epithelium. The reabsorptive mechanism utilises the sodium pump which extrudes the ion from the cell into the peritubular fluid. This allows sodium to pass into the cell from the lumen down a concentration gradient (Fig. 1.6).

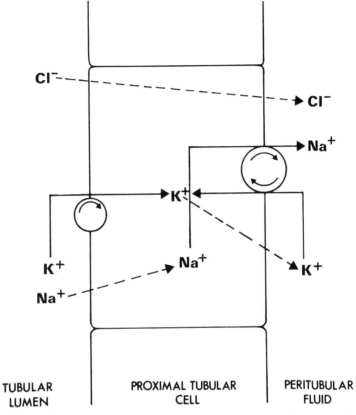

FIG. 1.6 Mechanism of electrolyte reabsorption in the proximal tubule.

PASSIVE REABSORPTION

The active reabsorption of sodium in the proximal tubule establishes gradients down which three other substances passively diffuse. An electrical gradient results in chloride reabsorption, an osmotic gradient that of water, and due to water reabsorption, a concentration gradient of urea builds up resulting in its reabsorption.

Renal handling of ions and water

At first sight, the system whereby large quantities of ions and water are filtered by the glomeruli and then mostly reabsorbed by the tubules seems inefficient. It is, however, the flexibility of this system which confers on the kidney the ability to maintain water and electrolyte balance even under extreme conditions. Table 1.1 shows the amount of ions and water being reabsorbed by the tubules each day, amounting to more than 99 per cent of filtered sodium, chloride, bicarbonate and water.

TABLE 1.1   Quantitative aspects of water and electrolyte handling.

	Quantity filtered (mmol/24 h)	Quantity excreted (mmol/24 h)	Per cent reabsorbed
Sodium	23 940	103	99·6
Chloride	19 845	103	99·5
Bicarbonate	5 103	2	> 99·9
Potassium	684	51	92·6
	(l/24 h)	(l/24 h)	
Water	169·2	1·5	99·1

THE PROXIMAL TUBULE

Reabsorption is isosmotic and within this segment 70–90 per cent of the glomerular filtrate is reabsorbed. The driving force is the sodium pump and the active removal of sodium from the tubular cell allows its entry from the lumen together with the passive reabsorption of chloride and water. Potassium is almost completely reabsorbed by a pump situated in the luminal border of the cell and there may also be active uptake from the peritubular fluid (Fig. 1.6).

THE LOOP OF HENLE

In contrast to the proximal tubule, salt is reabsorbed in excess of water, thus conserving salt and forming the basis for the countercurrent multiplier system (see below). Most of the active transport of salt takes place in the ascending limb and, again in contrast to the proximal tubule, is of chloride rather than sodium.

THE DISTAL TUBULE

While the proximal tubule reabsorbs most of the filtered ions and water in a fairly rigid manner, the distal tubule reabsorbs a much smaller fraction, probably 10 to 20 per cent, in a much more flexible way. The distal tubular cell is shown in Figure 1.7. As in the proximal tubule, sodium is extruded and potassium taken up by an active mechanism at the basal border of the cell and this regulates sodium uptake across the luminal border. Most of the movement of potassium across the luminal border is into the lumen down an electrical gradient created by the sodium uptake. Hydrogen ion moves in the same direction as potassium and there is an inverse

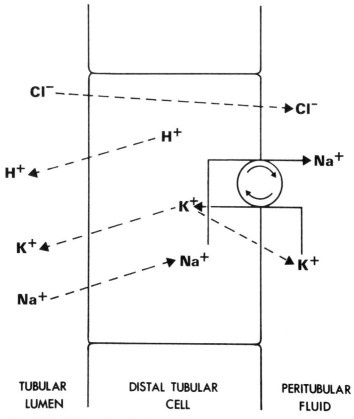

FIG. 1.7   Mechanism of electrolyte reabsorption in the distal tubule.

relationship between the movement of these two ions but no competition for a common pump, as has been suggested in the past. Chloride reabsorption is mainly passive although there is also evidence of an active transport mechanism as exists in the ascending limb. Finally, sodium reabsorption in the distal tubule is increased by aldosterone although it is often not appreciated that this hormone exhibits a similar though less powerful effect in the proximal tubule.

MECHANISM FOR WATER CONCENTRATION AND DILUTION

The concept of countercurrent multiplication has been proposed to explain the role of the loop of Henle and the hypertonic medulla in the production of a concentrated urine. This concept is illustrated in Figure 1.8 which depicts the ascending limb of the loop of Henle above and the descending limb below. An osmotic gradient is established between the distal and proximal limbs by active chloride reabsorption in the thick ascending limb. Although shown as a series of discontinuous steps, the fluid is constantly moving round the loop with isotonic fluid entering from the proximal tubule. The highest concentration is achieved at the bend of the loop while the fluid entering the distal tubule is hypotonic. For the system to work, the ascending thick limb must be impermeable to water. While the diagram shows the limbs in apposition, in the kidney they are separated by interstitial fluid. Figure 1.9 shows how the above principle can be applied to the kidney. The hypotonic fluid leaving Henle's loop traverses the distal tubule and enters the collecting duct. The permeability of the collecting duct wall to water is controlled by antidiuretic hormone (ADH). In the presence of water depletion, the increased permeability of the wall induced by ADH results in the reabsorption of water due to the osmotic effect of the hypertonic medulla, producing a concentrated urine. In states of fluid excess, the absence of ADH renders the collecting duct wall impermeable to water and the tubular fluid remains hypotonic, producing a dilute urine. The final part of the concept concerns the vasa recta, the long loops of capillaries which run in parallel to the loops of Henle. They form the countercurrent exchanger mechanism. As blood flows along these capillaries into the medulla, water diffuses out and solutes move in, so that the osmolality of the blood rises in parallel to that in the hypertonic

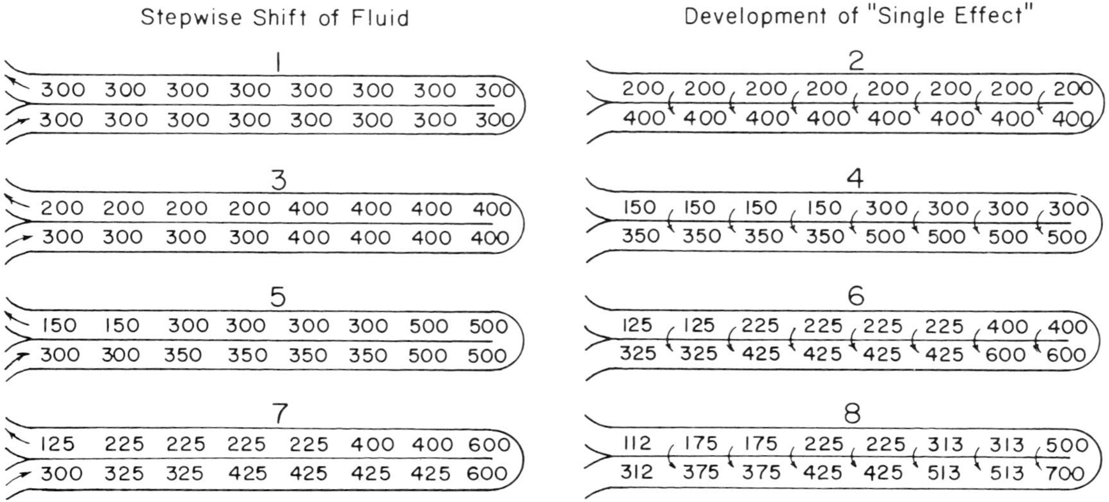

FIG. 1.8 Principle of the countercurrent multiplier system. An osmotic gradient is established between the ascending limb of the loop of Henle above and the descending limb below by active chloride reabsorption in the ascending limb. Reproduced with permission from Pitts, R. F. (1974) *Physiology of the Kidney and Body Fluids*, Chicago: Year Book.

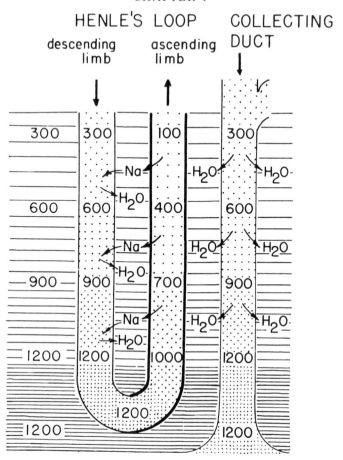

FIG. 1.9   Application of the countercurrent multiplier system to the kidney. The permeability of the collecting tubule to water is controlled by ADH. Reproduced with permission from Pitts, R. F. (1974) *Physiology of the Kidney and Body Fluids*, Chicago: Year Book.

interstitium. The reverse occurs as blood flows back into the cortex. This mechanism prevents dissipation of the hypertonicity built up by the countercurrent multiplier system.

Tubular secretion

The three types of tubular secretion are analogous to the three reabsorptive mechanisms.

TM LIMITED SECRETION

This type, in which there is an absolute limit to secretion similar to the reabsorption of glucose, is involved in the secretion of organic acids such as phenol red, PAH and penicillin and strong organic bases such as thiamine and histamine. The secretion of these compounds, many of which are foreign to the body, takes place in the proximal tubule.

GRADIENT TIME LIMITED SECRETION

Hydrogen ions are secreted by this mechanism against an electrochemical gradient in both the proximal and distal tubules. The previous suggestion that hydrogen and potassium compete for a common secretory pump in the distal tubule is now known to be incorrect, potassium being passively secreted down an electrical gradient.

PASSIVE SECRETION

In addition to potassium, substances secreted by this mechanism include weak bases such as ammonia and weak acids such as salicylic acid.

Regulation of acid–base balance

The bicarbonate–carbonic acid buffer system plays an essential role in acid–base balance. While the lungs remove large quantities of acid in the form of CO_2, the kidneys contribute in three ways, namely the conservation of bicarbonate, the excretion of acid in the form of ammonium salts, and the excretion of titratable acid. These three renal mechanisms are all dependent on the active secretion of hydrogen ion throughout the tubule.

REABSORPTION OF BICARBONATE

When acid–base balance is normal, more than 99·9 per cent of filtered bicarbonate is reabsorbed, 90 per cent in the proximal tubule and the remainder in the distal tubule. The mechanism is summarised in Figure 1.10. Hydrogen ion is actively secreted against an electrochemical gradient and combines with bicarbonate

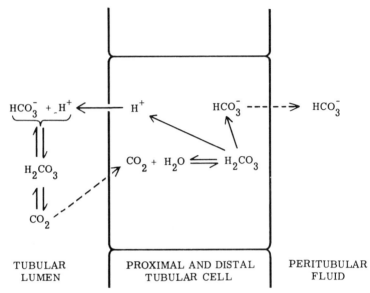

FIG. 1.10   Mechanism of reabsorption of bicarbonate, 90 per cent of which takes place in the proximal tubule and the remainder in the distal tubule.

in the tubular lumen. Carbonic acid is formed from which CO_2 is split off and reabsorbed to be hydrated and form carbonic acid again. This last step is dependent on the enzyme carbonic anhydrase. Bicarbonate reabsorption is virtually complete below a serum level of 28 mmol/l while increasing quantities appear in the urine as the plasma level rises above this value.

EXCRETION OF TITRATABLE ACID

This consists of the excretion of hydrogen ion in combination with buffers, of which phosphate is the most important. The mechanism is shown in Figure 1.11. Titratable acid represented by phosphate is formed mainly in the proximal tubule while that represented by other buffers such as β-hydroxybutyrate is formed mainly in the distal tubule.

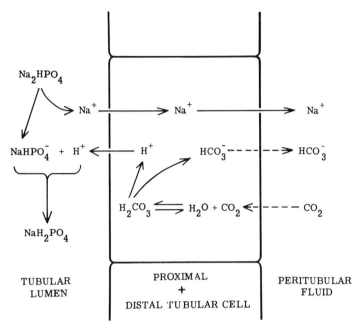

FIG. 1.11   Mechanism of excretion of titratable acid. Phosphate acts as a buffer mainly in the proximal tubule.

EXCRETION OF AMMONIA

Ammonia is formed in both proximal and distal tubular cells from a number of amino acids, in particular glutamine. The ammonia diffuses down a concentration gradient into the lumen where it combines with hydrogen to form the ammonium ion which is excreted mainly in the form of ammonium chloride (Fig. 1.12).

Under normal circumstances the kidney excretes 40–80 mmol of acid per day of which about 60 per cent combines with ammonia and the remainder is excreted as titratable acid.

Regulation of volume and osmolality of extracellular fluid

VOLUME

This is dependent on its sodium content. An increase of sodium causes thirst which results in the retention of water and therefore

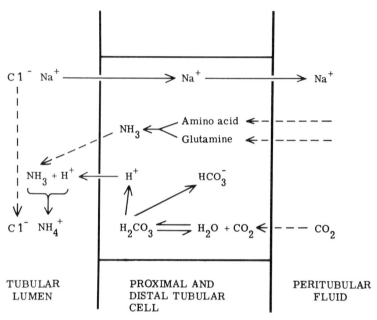

FIG. 1.12 Mechanism of excretion of acid in combination with ammonia. Ammonia is formed in both the proximal and distal tubule.

expansion of the extracellular fluid (ECF) volume. Two effector mechanisms will restore the volume to normal. One of these operates through volume receptors both inside and outside the vascular system which feed impulses to the hypothalamus. Thereafter there are several possible pathways which regulate the secretion of aldosterone and these are not mutually exclusive. The adrenal cortex can be stimulated by ADH directly, by ADH through the medium of ACTH, by the renin–angiotensin system and by adrenoglomerulotropin which is secreted by the diencephalon or pineal gland. When the ECF volume is increased, aldosterone secretion decreases under the influence of one or more of these regulatory pathways, urinary sodium excretion rises, and the ECF volume is restored to normal. The other mechanism also regulates sodium excretion but in this case directly. The increase in blood volume resulting from a sodium load has a direct haemodynamic effect in that renal blood flow and therefore glomerular filtration rate increases with a rise in the filtered load of sodium, leading to an increased urinary sodium loss.

OSMOLALITY

The osmolality of the ECF depends mainly on its water content and it is maintained within the range 283 ± 11 mosmol/kg by regulation of both intake and excretion of water. Osmoreceptors which are situated within the distribution of the internal carotid artery and possibly in the supraoptic nuclei detect changes in serum osmolality. An increase leads to thirst and to secretion of ADH by the posterior pituitary. Thirst has the effect of increasing the volume and reducing the osmolality of the ECF by increasing water intake. It is stimulated by a fall in ECF volume or rise in osmolality through an integrative centre in the hypothalamus. As discussed earlier, ADH increases water reabsorption in the collecting duct thus conserving water by production of a concentrated urine and tending to reduce the serum osmolality back to normal.

POINTS OF EMPHASIS

- At rest the RBF accounts for about 25 per cent of the cardiac output.

- The control of RBF involves both extrinsic and intrinsic mechanisms.

- A reduction in afferent arteriolar pressure causes an increase in renin release. This raises blood pressure and is also one of the factors which control RBF.

- Glomerular filtration is passive and largely depends upon molecular weight.

- Creatinine clearance provides a reasonably accurate guide of glomerular filtration rate.

- Both tubular reabsorption and secretion can be active or passive; the active mechanisms are either Tm limited or gradient time limited.

- All Tm limited reabsorption takes place in the proximal tubule.

- Sodium reabsorption in the proximal tubule is gradient time limited and is the main energy-consuming function of the kidney.

● From 70 to 90 per cent of the glomerular filtrate is reabsorbed in the proximal tubule. Most of the remainder, 10–20 per cent, is reabsorbed in a more flexible manner in the distal tubule.

● The production of a concentrated urine can be explained by the concept of a countercurrent multiplier system. Two important mechanisms are active chloride reabsorption in the ascending thick limb of Henle's loop which is impermeable to water, and the control of permeability to water of the collecting tubule by ADH.

● The kidney contributes to acid–base regulation by the reabsorption of bicarbonate and the excretion of ammonium salts and titratable acid, all three mechanisms depending upon the active secretion of hydrogen ion by the tubular cells.

CHAPTER 2

Clinical features and investigation of urinary tract disorders

Urinary tract symptoms

DYSURIA

This means pain on passing urine, often described as a burning sensation. It is usually due to bladder infection and, if so, is often associated with urgency which is the desire, often painful desire, to urinate. These two symptoms may also occur separately. Dysuria alone suggests inflammation of the urethra as occurs following cystoscopy or due to acute gonococcal urethritis. Urgency alone may be a pointer to neurological disease of the bladder. Closely related is the symptom of increased frequency of micturition, although the latter differs in that it does not imply discomfort. Increased frequency may be due either to bladder disease or an increased urine volume.

STRANGURY

This is severe, midline pain in the suprapubic region and radiating in men to the tip of the penis, due usually to a calculus in the urethra.

LOIN PAIN

There are two types of pain to consider (Fig. 2.1). The first is pain in the renal area, usually described as a dull aching pain, often radiating to the back and occurring in conditions such as a staghorn calculus or hydronephrosis. In acute pyelonephritis the pain is more intense and of acute onset. The other type of loin pain is ureteric colic which is spasmodic and radiates from the loin to the groin. It is

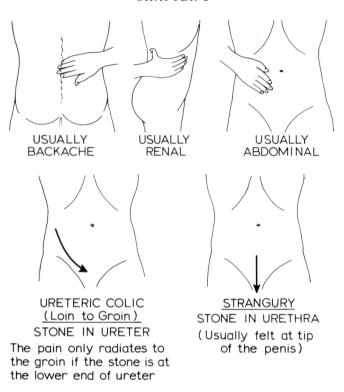

USUALLY
BACKACHE

USUALLY
RENAL

USUALLY
ABDOMINAL

URETERIC COLIC
(Loin to Groin)
STONE IN URETER
The pain only radiates to
the groin if the stone is at
the lower end of ureter

STRANGURY
STONE IN URETHRA
(Usually felt at tip
of the penis)

FIG. 2.1   The sites of the loin pain which occur in such conditions as hydronephrosis and acute pyelonephritis, the radiation of ureteric colic and the site of strangury.

usually due to a calculus or blood clot and typically the pain will radiate as far as the stone has travelled thus giving a guide to its position. Once the stone enters the bladder it is usually asymptomatic unless it then enters the urethra.

HAEMATURIA

This is an important symptom which, if confirmed by urine testing, justifies a thorough examination and investigation. It can be due to a wide range of diseases, some clues to which can be gained from the history. One distinction is between painful and painless haematuria. The former suggests infection or calculus and the latter a tumour. There may, of course, be a tumour and superimposed infection.

Blood from the upper urinary tract tends to be altered or brown, and that from the lower tract red. Blood appearing at the beginning of the urinary stream suggests an origin in the urethra. In medical conditions affecting the kidney, haematuria is frequent at a microscopic level but is not usually profuse enough to be noticed by the patient. Exceptions are acute glomerulonephritis with brown 'smoky' urine, focal glomerulonephritis with intermittent bright red blood, and polycystic kidneys which sometimes bleed giving rise also to loin pain.

Other urine abnormalities the patient may notice are an odour sometimes described as 'fishy', associated with a coliform urinary infection, and frothing which is an indication of heavy proteinuria.

INCONTINENCE

This is a deceptively difficult symptom to assess but is usually genuine even if special tests do not demonstrate it at the time of investigation. Some idea of the degree of incontinence can be obtained by asking what protection is required. Thus a patient who has to wear waterproof pants with many incontinence pads obviously has a severe problem whereas another may in fact have a small drip at the end of micturition which is overcome by remaining in the toilet a little longer. It is also true that people react to the degree of incontinence in different ways according to their personality. Thus a minor degree of incontinence can be very distressing to one particular patient whereas another may not even think it abnormal. Intermittent incontinence may be neurological in origin or secondary to an irritating bladder lesion (e.g. infection) or, especially in women, because of sphincter weakness. Continuous incontinence may be seen in association with overflow from a distended bladder or in patients with a fistula; most commonly a vesicovaginal fistula secondary to carcinoma of the cervix, radiotherapy or in undeveloped countries prolonged obstructed labour.

ENURESIS

This can be defined as nocturnal incontinence persisting after babyhood. Usually a child is dry at night by three years of age but there is considerable normal individual variation. Nocturnal incontinence persisting after the age of five years is referred to as primary enuresis. Nocturnal incontinence developing later in life is called secondary enuresis. Primary enuresis may be the result of a failure of the bladder to mature; such children have unstable bladders on cystometry (see Ch. 16). In other cases primary enuresis is attributed to deep sleep or more rarely psychological stress. Secondary enuresis may occur as a result of old age or neurological disease such as multiple sclerosis or nocturnal convulsions.

SYMPTOMS OF OBSTRUCTED MICTURITION

The classical symptom is a poor urinary stream: elderly men who are developing prostatic obstruction may find they have to spend longer and longer before completing micturition. The poor stream is often associated with hesitancy and this is typically worst shortly after rising in the morning. There is also associated post-micturition dribbling and urinary spray; these symptoms arise from the distortion an enlarged prostate causes to the urethra. Increased frequency of micturition or urgency are often superimposed on those of obstruction but these are due to bladder irritability rather than the obstruction itself. The force of the stream can often be best assessed in men by asking how near they have to stand to the toilet.

NOCTURIA

This is the need to rise at night to pass urine and may range from once to several times. It may indicate impairment of renal function resulting in polyuria and loss of the normal diurnal rhythm of urine flow, or it may indicate a change in bladder function of which the commonest causes are instability in women or prostatic obstruction in older men.

POLYURIA

This is an increase in the 24-hour urine volume. It is due either to the impaired ability of a damaged kidney to produce a concentrated urine or to an increased solute load as in diabetes mellitus. In common with nocturia, this symptom is seldom reported spontaneously, but while the patient finds nocturia easy to recognise, the response to enquiry about polyuria may be vague.

PNEUMATURIA

This bizarre symptom is usually accurately described by the patient as a sensation of passing bubbles in the urine. There may be a history of associated passage of faeculant material. The commonest cause is fistula into the bladder usually secondary to diverticular disease or carcinoma of the large bowel. A much rarer cause is fermentation of the urine in a case of diabetes the so-called 'illicit still syndrome'.

Examination

General examination of the patient may reveal some pointers to urinary tract disease. For example, it should be remembered that confusion in an elderly man may be the result of uraemia from chronic bladder obstruction by a large prostate. Other features of uraemia may inlude a sallow complexion, scratch marks (due to itch), a coarse tremor, acidotic respiration, hiccoughs, pericardial friction and rarely small deposits of urea crystals on the skin, so called uraemic frost. All these features are usually seen only in advanced uraemia.

Examination of the abdomen consists of inspection, percussion, palpation and auscultation. Inspection may reveal a lower abdominal swelling with an enlarged bladder. Retroperitoneal masses and renal masses are more difficult to feel and are not usually evident on inspection except occasionally in children. Palpation for renal masses is carried out with both hands. It is usual in a thin person to be able to feel the lower pole of the right kidney and sometimes the left kidney which lies slightly higher. Percussion is useful to determine bladder enlargement particularly in the obese patient when palpation may be difficult. Rectal examination is a routine part of any abdominal examination. In a man the prostate is carefully palpated and it is noted whether the consistency is rubbery (i.e. benign) or hard (i.e. possibly malignant). In addition to the consistency, the contour of the prostate is felt. The two lateral lobes are usually palpable with a median groove. Carcinoma of the prostate may distort this contour. Auscultation is not particularly helpful in urological patients although occasionally renal artery bruits may be heard in patients with hypertension secondary to renal artery stenosis. Patients with suspected abdominal

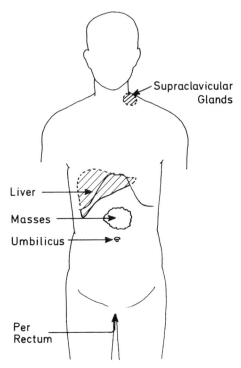

FIG. 2.2   Physical examination to detect secondary spread from intra-abdominal primary cancer.

malignancy should have a thorough inspection for glandular metastases (Fig. 2.2).

Investigation

PROTEINURIA

Urine testing for protein should form part of every medical examination even if renal disease is not suspected. The stick test (e.g. Albustix or Multistix, Ames Company Ltd) is very sensitive and occasional positive results are recorded in normal subjects. Thus unexpected positive results should be checked by boiling acidified urine or adding 25 per cent sulphosalicylic acid. Once proteinuria has been confirmed, a quantitative measurement should be carried out on a 24-hour urine collection. A result over

150 mg per day is abnormal, and over two grams per day usually indicates glomerular disease. Occasionally in young adults proteinuria is orthostatic (or postural), i.e. present only when in the upright position. This condition is rarely of significance and can be diagnosed by comparing urine samples obtained when the individual is fully recumbent and when up and about.

URINE MICROSCOPY

This should be carried out routinely and with care. A fairly simple but accurate method consists of centrifugation at 500 rpm of a random 10 ml sample with removal of the top 9·5 ml and re-suspension of the sediment in the remaining 0·5 ml. An aliquot of this is placed in a Nebauer counting chamber and all the cells in one of the five vertical columns in the central part of the chamber are counted. More than five red or white cells are abnormal. Microscopic haematuria occurs in a wide variety of renal diseases but determination of its presence can have considerable diagnostic value.

URINE CULTURE

The mid-stream urine sample (MSU) is the standard method but has the disadvantage of the presence of at least a few contaminant organisms even with good technique. For this reason, quantitation of urine organisms should be a routine technique. Contaminants usually number less than 10000 bacteria per millilitre whereas more than 100000 organisms per millilitre indicates a significant infection. The aspiration of bladder urine by suprapubic puncture avoids the problem of contamination but the greater complexity and trauma to the patient, although slight, do not justify its routine use. It does, however, have a place in infancy where an MSU is difficult to obtain. Urine culture can be performed by conventional methods but the use of dipslides (Fig. 2.3) has the two important advantages of allowing transportation of the samples and saving time in the laboratory.

GLOMERULAR FILTRATION RATE

Blood urea has been widely used as an indirect measure of GFR and, while its main determinant is the GFR, it is only a crude

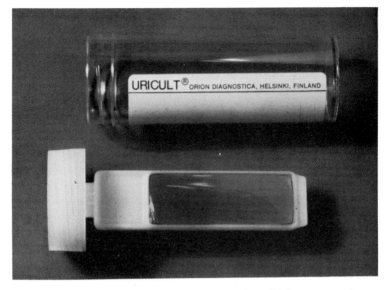

FIG. 2.3 The dipslide consists of a culture plate with its own container which can either be dipped in the urine sample or held in the urinary stream. The colonies are then counted in the laboratory after the appropriate period of incubation.

measure because of other influences such as the rate of protein breakdown and the state of hydration. The upper limit of normal is 6 mmol/l. The serum creatinine more accurately reflects GFR although a transient rise follows ingestion of cooked meat. The creatinine clearance is widely used for measurement of GFR in routine clinical practice while more accurate methods utilise isotopes such as ^{131}I Hypaque and ^{51}Cr EDTA. The results should be related to body surface area.

SERUM ELECTROLYTES

These give a wide range of information relating to more than renal function; Table 2.1 lists some of the commoner abnormalities. This subject is discussed in Chapter 5.

URINE CONCENTRATING POWER

This is a simple test of overall tubular function but is seldom

TABLE 2.1   Serum electrolytes.

	Low	High
Sodium	(Hyponatraemia: <130 mmol/l) 1. Na$^+$ depletion 2. Generalised oedema 3. Secondary hyperaldosteronism 4. Inappropriate ADH secretion 5. Sick cell syndrome	(Hypernatraemia: >145 mmol/l) 1. Water depletion 2. Excess sodium administration, e.g. in coma
Potassium	(Hypokalaemia: <3·5 mmol/l) 1. K$^+$ depletion 2. Alkalosis	(Hyperkalaemia: >5·5 mmol/l) 1. Oliguria 2. Tissue damage 3. Acidosis 4. Adrenal insufficiency
Chloride	(Hypochloraemia: <95 mmol/l) 1. Cl$^-$ depletion 2. Alkalosis	(Hyperchloraemia: >110 mmol/l) 1. Water depletion 2. Acidosis (renal tubular acidosis or lower gastrointestinal fluid loss)
Bicarbonate	(Metabolic acidosis: <24 mmol/l) 1. Renal failure 2. Diabetic ketoacidosis 3. Lactic acidosis 4. Toxins, e.g. salicylates	(Metabolic alkalosis: >30 mmol/l) 1. Alkali ingestion 2. Upper gastrointestinal fluid loss 3. Diuretics 4. Hyperaldosteronism or increased mineralo-corticoid production

of diagnostic help other than in suspected diabetes insipidus. Either the intramuscular injection of pitressin in oil (5 units) or withholding fluid for 18 hours should result in a urine osmolality of more than 800 mosmol/kg.

URINARY ACIDIFICATION

Tests of this aspect of renal function are used mainly in the diagnosis of renal tubular acidosis (RTA). In this condition, unlike chronic renal failure, the urine pH remains above 5·4 even in the presence of systemic acidosis (see Chapter 5).

RADIOLOGY

Plain film. The purpose of this is to detect renal calcification and calculi. It forms a preliminary to an intravenous urogram (IVU) but is also of value on its own in the follow-up of patients with calculous disease.

Intravenous urogram. The standard way of visualising renal anatomy is by the IVU. Various iodine-containing contrast media are used as sodium or meglumine salts; sodium is more popular. The standard dose of iodine is 300 mg/kg body weight, equivalent to 1 ml/kg of most preparations. Doubling of the dose is necessary to provide useful information in renal failure. It is important that the patient is adequately prepared by dehydration to give a greater concentration of contrast medium. The exception to this is in renal failure where it is potentially harmful. A test dose of the medium should be given to reduce the risk of severe hypersensitivity reactions. The main injection is then given and an immediate film taken which should show the renal outlines and parenchymal thickness. Further films are obtained during the next 15 minutes to give visualisation of the collecting system. Prior to these films a compression band can be put across the abdomen to delay the passage of contrast down the ureter and thus give improved definition of the renal pelvis and calyces. The compression band is then released and a full length film is taken to display the whole ureter from kidney to bladder. A separate film is taken of the bladder area to obtain more precise detail of the lower ends of the ureters and bladder size. Finally, it is helpful in many cases to repeat the film of the bladder area after voiding to see if there is any residual urine. The use of tomography will improve definition particularly of the renal outlines and is indicated in renal failure, or when there is inadequate dehydration or considerable overlying gas in the bowel. Comprehensive examination of an IVU can yield much useful information, as shown in Table 2.2. The IVU can still give useful diagnostic information when renal function is very poor in both acute and chronic renal failure (see Ch. 8 and 9).

Retrograde ureterogram and pyelogram. These are radiological

TABLE 2.2 Intravenous urogram.

Component	Diagnostic value
Plain film	Nephrocalcinosis (hypercalcaemia, renal tubular acidosis, medullary sponge kidney, hyperoxaluria) Calcification of tuberculosis Papillary calcification (papillary necrosis) Calculi in kidney, ureter or bladder
Renal outline	Bipolar length Cortical scarring (solitary or multiple) Localised swelling (single, e.g. cyst or tumour; multiple, e.g. cysts)
Calyces	Dilatation (focal, e.g. pyelonephritis; generalised, e.g. obstruction) Papillary necrosis (phenacetin habituation, tuberculosis) Compression (cyst or tumour)
Pelvis	Dilatation (hydronephrosis) Filling defect (papilloma)
Ureter	Dilatation (hydroureter) Stricture Displacement (tumour or retroperitoneal fibrosis)
Bladder	Dilatation (obstruction or neurological disease) Contraction (chronic inflammation, e.g. tuberculosis) Filling defects (tumours or calculi)
Miscellaneous	Comparison of rate of excretion of contrast (unequal in renal artery stenosis)

investigations where contrast is injected up a ureteric catheter and their main value is to determine the position of any ureteric obstruction. An ascending ureterogram is a variation where contrast is injected up the ureter through a catheter held against the ureteric orifice. This examination must be performed on the X-ray table and is only practical where facilities exist for image intensification.

Antegrade pyelogram. If dilated, the renal pelvis or a calyx can be punctured by a needle inserted percutaneously (usually under ultrasound control) and contrast injected. This investigation is useful where there is poor renal function, making intravenous pyelography impossible and where retrograde or ascending ureterograms also prove impossible, e.g. when a pelvic tumour is distorting the bladder and obscuring the ureteric orifices.

Micturating cystogram. This is an X-ray of the bladder during filling and voiding. The catheter is then removed. A urethral catheter is passed and the bladder is filled with contrast. Films are taken to show the bladder shape and size; alteration of shape may be characteristic, e.g. the 'fir tree' shape is characteristic of many neurogenic bladders. Further films are taken during voiding and these will show whether any urine refluxes up the ureters and whether urine flows freely through the bladder neck into the urethra.

Urethrogram. An ascending urethrogram is used to define urethral lesions such as a stricture. Viscous radio-opaque jelly is injected through the penile meatus. Strictures in the prostatic area are better defined by a descending urethrogram. Contrast is introduced into the bladder through a fine catheter and pictures taken during attempts to void.

Arteriogram. An IVU may reveal certain abnormalities which require further investigation. One approach is by arteriography. This is an invasive investigation which carries some risk of arterial damage and embolisation into the legs. Contrast medium is injected through a catheter passed up the femoral artery into the aorta (ileo-femoral approach). Should extensive atheroma preclude this approach, direct puncture of the abdominal aorta can be performed by a needle inserted into the lumbar region (translumbar approach). When the ileo-femoral approach is used, the catheter may be placed in the aorta (non-selective technique) or in the renal artery itself (selective technique).

The main indication is the need to provide further information about vascular lesions such as arterial stenosis, aneurysm and thrombosis. The simpler technique of ultrasound can usually differentiate cysts from tumours but arteriography may be required in the case of a suspected tumour to demonstrate its extent and vascular anatomy. In addition to confirming the diagnosis of renal artery stenosis, arteriography with the aid of a special catheter can now be used to dilate the stenotic segment. Finally, the arteriogram can be helpful in the localisation of profuse bleeding following trauma or biopsy. Following localisation, it may be possible to selectively embolise the bleeding vessels and thus stop the haemorrhage by producing a localised infarct. This involves injecting a variety of substances such as autologous blood coagulated with epsilon amino caproic acid. This technique of embolisation is also being used increasingly prior to surgery to reduce blood loss.

Ultrasound examination. This can be of considerable diagnostic value under the following circumstances:

1. When an IVU shows a space-occupying lesion, ultrasound can differentiate a cyst from a solid tumour. Occasionally, a renal carcinoma is cystic and therefore when a cystic lesion is detected it is standard practice to aspirate the cyst under ultrasound control. The mass is dismissed as benign only if it disappears completely after aspiration and the fluid is negative on cytological examination for malignant cells.

2. It is useful in the diagnosis of hydronephrosis particularly when there is poor or absent visualisation on the IVU. It will differentiate clearly the hydronephrotic from the small, contracted kidney in chronic renal failure.

3. It is a simple and reliable method of screening families for polycystic kidneys.

4. Localisation of the kidney for percutaneous biopsy is easily and accurately performed with ultrasound.

Isotope studies. Renal scanning is also a non-invasive investigation. Table 2.3 indicates the application of isotope methods to the investigation of the urinary tract. Renal plasma flow (RPF) and glomerular filtration rate (GFR) can be measured using a constant infusion or more simply by a single injection with several blood samples. Modern scanning equipment usually includes a gamma camera linked to a computer and the most suitable isotope is

TABLE 2.3   Isotope studies.

Technique	Isotope
Measurement of renal plasma flow	^{123}I or ^{131}I Hippuran
Measurement of glomerular filtration rate	^{131}I Hypaque or ^{51}Cr EDTA
Gamma camera renography	^{123}I or ^{131}I Hippuran Technetium-labelled DTPA Technetium-labelled DMSA Technetium

¹²³I Hippuran. This provides polaroid pictures for anatomical information and also a time/activity curve (Fig. 2.4). The latter shows the renal transit time of the isotope which is useful in the diagnosis of renal artery stenosis and urinary tract obstruction. Simultaneous blood sampling allows measurement of RPF as well. The use of ¹²³I gives a much lower radiation dose than ¹³¹I but is not so widely available. Diethylene triamine penta-acetic acid (DTPA) labelled with technetium is excreted by glomerular filtration and is

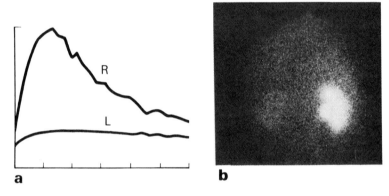

a   b

Fig. 2.4   (a) A time-activity curve using ¹²³Hippuran showing the right kidney (R) to have a normal pattern while the left kidney (L) has very poor function.
(b) A gamma camera photograph showing the smaller left kidney with poor isotope excretion.

an alternative for renography. Dimercapto-succinic acid (DMSA), also labelled with technetium, is taken up and retained by the renal tubules. The resultant gamma camera picture gives a good idea of the renal outline and parenchymal thickness and in fact this technique is superior to the IVU in localising early functional cortical loss, particularly if this is patchy. Later pictures can be taken as the nucleotide collects in the renal pelvis and passes down the ureter. Technetium in the free form can be used as a measure of renal perfusion even in the absence of kidney function as in acute tubular necrosis. It is therefore of value in the assessment of renal perfusion shortly after transplantation if the onset of renal function is delayed. The dose of radiation from renal scanning is about one-third that of a conventional IVU and it is of particular value in the follow-up of patients who would otherwise require repeated IVUs, e.g. a patient with obstruction from a ureteric stricture.

Cystoscopy and urethroscopy. These are used to examine the anatomy of the urethra and bladder. The cystoscope is essentially a smooth tube that can be passed through the urethra and various telescopes allow inspection of the bladder and urethra. As a general rule a cystoscope should never be passed without the opportunity being taken to inspect the urethra as well as the bladder. Urethral strictures can be incised, bladder tumours treated with diathermy and bladder stones manipulated under direct vision using instruments passed through the cystoscope. Cystoscopy is usually performed under general anaesthesia.

Ureteric catheterisation. The ureteric orifice is easily seen during cytoscopic examination. Ureteric catheters may be passed for several reasons apart from the injection of contrast:

1. To collect urine from each kidney for differential renal function studies; modern renography is making this investigation obsolete.
2. To collect organisms from a suspected tuberculous kidney.
3. To collect epithelial cells from a possible tumour in the renal pelvis.
4. To effect drainage where there is an obstruction to urine flow.

Cystometry is often combined with micturating cystography to further assess bladder function. It is an investigation where the bladder pressure is measured during filling and voiding (see Ch. 16). Pressure may also be measured in the urethra—the urethral pressure profile. Cystometry and urethral pressure profiles are particularly useful to assess incontinence and it is now true to say that no woman should undergo a gynaecological repair operation without first having these investigations done to make sure that a weak urethra is indeed the cause of her symptoms.

RENAL BIOPSY

The indications are:

1. Proteinuria of more than 1 g/24 h.

2. Unexplained renal failure in association with normal renal size.
3. Haematuria where both the IVU and lower urinary tract are normal.
4. Abnormal urinary sediment in association with multisystem disease, e.g. systemic lupus erythematosus.
5. Following renal transplantation to confirm severe rejection.

Before performing a biopsy, it should be confirmed that blood coagulation tests are normal, hypertension is controlled and that both kidneys are present and not markedly shrunken. The patient's blood group should be determined and two units of blood should be cross-matched and held in reserve. Prior localisation of the kidneys utilising an IVU and ultrasound is also helpful to assess the depth from the skin surface. With the patient lying prone or sitting and under local anaesthesia, a modified Vim–Silverman or disposable Travenol Tru-Cut biopsy needle is inserted into either kidney below the twelfth rib. Positioning of the needle during the procedure can be aided by an X-ray with injection of contrast medium or by ultrasound. Such aids during the procedure are, however, not essential. Following the biopsy, the patient should remain recumbent for 24 hours with blood pressure recordings during the first few hours. The main complicaton is bleeding either in the form of haematuria or perinephric haematoma. Minor degrees of bleeding are very frequent but major haemorrhage is unusual. Two cores of renal tissue are usually obtained which are divided up and processed for examination by light, fluorescence and electron microscopy.

POINTS OF EMPHASIS

● Haematuria is an important symptom which demands thorough investigation.

● The features of uraemia are often non-specific and present only at a late stage.

● It is usual to feel the lower pole of the right kidney in a thin subject.

● Rectal examination to assess the size and consistency of the prostate should be performed as a routine.

● Urine testing for proteinuria should be part of every medical examination.

● Proteinuria in excess of 2 g/24 h usually indicates glomerular disease.

● An IVU examination should be preceded by dehydration except in renal failure when this is potentially dangerous. Elderly patients should also be dehydrated with care.

● The IVU with tomography can give useful diagnostic information even when renal function is very poor.

● The main indication for retrograde pyelography is to confirm and localise ureteric obstruction.

● Arteriography is not without risk but can be helpful in the diagnosis of vascular lesions and also of therapeutic value to produce embolisation in cases of profuse haemorrhage.

● Ultrasound is of special value in distinguishing a cystic lesion from a solid tumour.

● Renal scanning may provide greater functional information than an IVU at about a third of the dose of radiation.

● The indications for renal biopsy include significant proteinuria, haematuria, unexplained renal failure with normal renal size and an abnormal urinary sediment in association with multisystem disease.

CHAPTER 3

Congenital and inherited disorders of the renal tract

INTRODUCTION

All classifications used to present this subject are necessarily arbitrary because our knowledge of many of the conditions is limited. Many are rare; some present in adult life and others may only be discovered accidentally. Some syndromes have more than one name and others may contain many subgroups which have yet to be differentiated. In all, the aetiology and pathogenesis is unclear.

CONGENITAL DISORDERS OF DEVELOPMENT

Renal agenesis
Complete failure of development of one kidney occurs quite commonly (about 1 in 2000 of the general population). No clinical consequences ensue providing the remaining kidney is normal. However, any disease or injury to that kidney carries the threat of renal failure. There is often an associated absence of the vas deferens on the same side.

Renal hypoplasia

A hypoplastic kidney has a diminished number of renal lobes. The kidney is smaller, has fewer calyces and nephrons, but is otherwise normal. These features may be defined by intravenous urography.

UNILATERAL HYPOPLASIA

This occurs in about 1 in 500 of the adult population. There is some evidence that it may lead to recurrent infection, stone formation and hypertension in a minority of affected individuals.

SEGMENTAL HYPOPLASIA

If only part of the kidney is involved, the renal outline may be depressed and the underlying calyx deformed. Therefore, the radiological features are very similar to those of chronic pyelonephritis (see Ch. 4) especially as the anatomical abnormality may lead to infection and hypertension. On histological examination, however, the hypoplastic area contains a reduced number of glomeruli surrounded by atrophic tubules.

BILATERAL HYPOPLASIA

Bilateral hypoplasia is a cause of renal insufficiency which may be progressive and is a relatively common cause of terminal renal failure in childhood. Renal hypoplasia is often associated with abnormalities of the central nervous system, and the children are often small for their age. It is also seen as part of some inherited syndromes, e.g. the 13q-syndrome.

OLIGOMEGANEPHRONIA

This is a rare congenital abnormality in which the total number of nephrons is only 20 per cent of the normal number, but they are all grossly enlarged. However, the overall size of the kidney is reduced. The patients present with evidence of tubular dysfunction such as polyuria or hyperchloraemic acidosis. Progressive renal failure usually develops and most children die in late childhood.

Renal dysplasia

A dysplastic kidney is the result of defective structural differentiation of the metanephros. This may result in cystic or solid abnormalities and commonly coexists with renal hypoplasia. Most are associated with abnormalities of the ureter, bladder or urethra. Therefore, it is possible that urinary tract obstruction during development of the kidney may be the cause of these abnormalities. Histological abnormalities include plaques of cartilage in the cortex and primitive ducts in the medulla. Cysts are common and may be very large. The dysplastic segment is non-functioning. If both kidneys are severely affected, the infant is stillborn. Unilateral disease may lead to hypertension, loin pain, infections and stone formation—all of which may appear at any age, and may be an indication for nephrectomy.

Cystic renal dysplasia is usually found without evidence of other congenital disorders but may be associated with several rare syndromes.

Medullary sponge kidney

The basic abnormality of this syndrome is ectasia of the distal portion of the collecting ducts. Cysts, lined with columnar or transitional cells, develop in the renal papilla. These cysts are filled with gelatinous material in which stones develop. Although the abnormality is congenital, patients usually present between the ages of 20 and 50 with renal colic, haematuria or urinary tract infection. Tubular abnormalities, such as failure to acidify the urine normally and hypercalcuria, are sometimes found. Twenty per cent of patients have other congenital abnormalities. Occasionally more than one member of a family is affected and it is found predominately in males.

The diagnosis is made by the appearance of the intravenous urogram. On the plain film, small clusters of stones are seen in the region of the papillae. The kidneys are normal or slightly enlarged in size and ductal ectasia may be demonstrated in later films.

The prognosis is excellent although periodic symptoms occur throughout life.

INHERITED CYSTIC DISORDERS OF DEVELOPMENT

Infantile polycystic kidneys

This is a rare condition inherited as an autosomal recessive. Clinical presentations are:

1. Obstructed labour due to the large size of the kidneys and death in the perinatal period from uraemia or respiratory failure. This is the most common type.
2. Most survivors of the perinatal period die within the first year with hypertension, heart failure and progressive renal failure.
3. A very few survive to adolescence when they develop portal hypertension due to hepatic fibrosis.

PATHOLOGY

The kidneys are often huge, particularly in those who die at birth, in whom they may be 12 times the normal size. The surface is smooth, but the kidney is made up of elongated cysts arranged radially and lined by cuboidal epithelium. The glomeruli appear to be reduced in number and are grossly dilated. In patients surviving to adolescence, fewer nephrons are affected. The cause of these gross abnormalities is unknown but may be due to tubular injury during development.

Adult polycystic kidneys

INCIDENCE

Dalgaard estimated that 1 in 3500 of the general population suffer from this disorder. It is somewhat more common in post mortem series, varying between 1 in 222 and 1 in 1010. Eight per cent of the patients taken on to the dialysis programmes of Europe have polycystic renal disease.

INHERITANCE

It is inherited as an autosomal dominant, but about 30 per cent of patients have no apparent family history. Males and females are affected in equal numbers.

AGE OF ONSET

Symptoms develop most frequently between the ages of 25 to 35 and renal failure progresses over the next 10 to 15 years. Each patient tends to run a similar time course to other affected members of his family.

PATHOLOGY

Both kidneys are affected but one may be conspicuously more enlarged than the other. Cysts develop in any part of the nephron. They are found in both cortex and medulla and progressively increase in size. The largest may be up to 5 cm in diameter. Strands of normal parenchyma persist around and between the cysts, although evidence of pyelonephritis, calcification and hypertension may be apparent. Bleeding into the cysts also occurs. When terminal renal failure sets in, the kidneys are huge, weighing up to ten times normal. Cysts are also found in the liver (30 per cent), pancreas (ten per cent) and 15 per cent of patients have berry aneurysms of the Circle of Willis.

CLINICAL PRESENTATION

The condition may be diagnosed when the patient feels an abdominal fullness or accidentally when the abdomen is examined for some other reason. More commonly, urinary infection, haematuria or the development of renal failure draw attention to the diagnosis. Hypertension is a rarer presentation.

The clinical course is one of slow progress to renal failure. Hypertension develops in 50 per cent of patients but is usually easily controlled. Anaemia is less marked than in other causes of renal failure. The patient may suffer periodic episodes of loin pain due to infection or haemorrhage into a cyst. Renal calculi may form but rarely give rise to symptoms.

Subarachnoid haemorrhages may occur at any time and are the cause of ten per cent of deaths. The cysts in the liver and pancreas rarely cause any symptoms. Fifty per cent of patients develop terminal renal failure, ten per cent die of congestive cardiac failure and ten per cent of myocardial infarcts. Very occasionally, a malignancy may develop in one of the kidneys.

DIAGNOSIS

The finding of bilateral loin masses, on which discrete cysts can often be felt, is pathognomonic of polycystic renal disease. Intravenous urography is a more common way of making the diagnosis. Both kidneys are large, the outer surfaces of the kidneys cannot always be clearly demarcated and the calyceal system is grossly distorted as the calyces are stretched around the cysts. A calyx may appear narrow and attenuated if viewed in profile and broad if viewed *en face*. Ultrasound examination of the kidney is a useful way of detecting enlargement of the kidney and the presence of transonic cysts.

TREATMENT

No specific treatment exists. Blood pressure should be rigorously controlled and this may lower the incidence of subarachnoid haemorrhage. Infection should be treated. There is little place for cyst puncture (Rovsing's procedure) which at one time was thought to slow the development of renal failure. Occasionally severe pain or ureteric compression may be relieved by surgical decompression of a cyst. Most patients who develop terminal renal failure are suitable for dialysis and transplantation. Bilateral nephrectomies may be necessary in patients who have huge kidneys (in order to make room for the transplant) or who have had recurrent infection as immunosuppressive therapy may precipitate disseminated infection.

Genetic counselling should be offered to all patients in whom the diagnosis is made before they have children and for this reason an attempt should also be made to diagnose affected offspring. This may be best achieved by ultrasound examination of the kidney performed soon after the 20th birthday. The relatives of affected individuals should also be screened for hypertension.

Medullary cystic disease and juvenile nephronophthisis

These may be two names for the same disease but there are some distinguishing features.

INHERITANCE

Both appear sporadically, but juvenile nephronophthisis is probably inherited as an autosomal recessive and medullary cystic disease as an autosomal dominant.

PATHOLOGY

The two conditions cannot be distinguished at autopsy. The kidneys are smooth and small and the cortex is thin. The medulla is usually replaced by numerous cysts. Microdissection reveals that the cysts arise from the collecting ducts and distal tubules. Cysts are not found in every patient but gross interstitial inflammation is found in the medulla of all patients.

AGE OF ONSET

Juvenile nephronophthisis presents in childhood and accounts for 10–20 per cent of children with renal failure. Medullary cystic disease most commonly presents in the third decade. Both sexes are equally affected.

CLINICAL COURSE

Both present with polyuria and polydipsia; anaemia, often out of proportion to the degree of renal failure, is common. Many children are small for their age. Hypertension develops in 30 per cent and renal failure is progressive in all, usually being terminal within four years of diagnosis.

Juvenile nephronophthisis is sometimes associated with extrarenal manifestations, such as retinal and cerebellar degeneration, mental retardation and some skeletal abnormalities.

TREATMENT

No specific treatment exists. Hypokalaemia may require correction with potassium supplements, but dialysis and transplantation offer the only hope of long term survival.

HEREDITARY CHRONIC NEPHRITIS

Alport's syndrome

This is the association of nephritis and deafness.

INHERITANCE

The disease affects both sexes but it is much more severe in males. Affected fathers rarely transmit the disease to their sons. The exact mode of transmission remains in doubt. It may be as a partial sex-linked dominant, or autosomal dominant (in which case other factors, perhaps hormonal, would need to be postulated to account for the sex variation), or by preferential segregation of the affected chromosome with the X chromosome in males.

PATHOLOGY

The kidneys become smaller as the disease progresses but scars do not develop. The glomeruli show changes of mesangial proliferation and some crescent formation. Tubular atrophy and interstitial infiltrate including foam cells occur, sometimes independently of the glomerular changes. On electron microscopic examination of the glomeruli, the lamina densa of the basement membrane is split and laminated. Immunofluorescent studies of the glomeruli show IgM and C3 deposition in areas of sclerosis.

CLINICAL COURSE

Males are affected earlier and more severely than females. Symptoms usually develop in the second decade in males. Episodes of haematuria, often following infections of the respiratory tract, are common. Proteinuria is usually not severe although occasionally it may be of sufficient extent to cause the nephrotic syndrome. Slowly progressive renal failure is the rule in males, who develop terminal renal failure before the age of 40. Hypertension is common.

Women rarely develop severe renal failure, but may have episodes of haematuria following stress or during pregnancy.

Deafness is common and starts with bilateral loss of high frequency acuity, which may only be detectable on audiography early in the disease. Its rate of progress is variable, some patients ultimately having severe deafness. Ocular manifestations occur in 15 per cent of patients. Again males are affected more commonly by cataracts, lenticonus, spherophakia and retinitis pigmentosa.

TREATMENT

No specific treatment exists; patients are usually suitable for dialysis and/or transplantation.

Familial recurrent haematuria

This is a benign disease characterised by episodes of frank haematuria often following minor upper respiratory tract infections in a patient who is otherwise well. The prognosis is excellent. It may occur sporadically or be inherited as an autosomal dominant or recessive.

Nail patella syndrome (Hereditary onycho-osteodysplasia)

This syndrome comprises dystrophic and hypoplastic nails, iliac horns, hypoplastic patellae and malformation of the head of the radius. Some patients have an abnormality of the pigment of the iris and/or deafness. Renal involvement, which takes the form of proteinuria, occurs in 30–40 per cent. Of those with renal involvement, 25 per cent develop progressive renal failure.

INHERITANCE

The condition is inherited as an autosomal dominant.

PATHOLOGY

The glomerular basement membrane is irregularly thickened and contains lucent areas which are irregularly distributed. Collagen fibres can be demonstrated within the GBM by electron microscopy.

TREATMENT

There is no specific therapy.

Angiokeratoma corporis diffusum (Fabry's disease)

This is a rare inherited disorder of lipid metabolism due to a lack of the enzyme ceramide trihexosidase. This leads to deposition of ceramide trihexoside and ceramide dihexoside in the skin, kidney, nervous system and cardiovascular system.

INHERITANCE

Males are affected more severely, but females are carriers. Thus an incompletely recessive X-linked gene is postulated.

PATHOLOGY

The cells of the glomerular tuft and distal tubules are filled with deposits of lipids, which appear as vacuoles on light microscopy and foamy material on electron microscopy.

CLINICAL COURSE

The onset usually occurs in childhood at the age of 9 or 10. Dark red spots about 2 cm in diameter develop on the skin, particularly over the buttocks and lumbar region. These angiomas slowly progress. Episodes of fever, paraesthesia, excrutiating pains in the limbs and abdominal colic occur and may pre-date the rash thus making diagnosis very difficult. Proteinuria may also be present. After a few years, these attacks become less frequent and the only evidence of the disease is the skin angiomas. In early adult life renal failure with hypertension develops and death occurs by the age of 40.

TREATMENT

No specific therapy exists; attempts to transfuse the missing enzyme (ceramide trihexosidase) by various methods have been largely unsuccessful. Dialysis and transplantation is often successful and the transplanted kidney may be a source of the missing enzyme.

Familial Mediterranean fever

This is a genetic disorder occurring most frequently in Sephardic Jews and Armenians. There are two principal clinical manifestations. Acute attacks consisting of fever, peritonitis, pleuritis, synovitis and an erysipelas-like erythema appear first. They are self-limiting, usually only lasting a few days, although synovitis may persist for longer. The second major clinical manifestation is amyloidosis which is deposited in the spleen, liver, adrenals and kidneys. Renal involvement starts with proteinuria, and the nephrotic syndrome and progressive renal failure develop. Most patients die or are on dialysis by the age of 40. Amyloid deposition in other organs apparently produces few symptoms.

TREATMENT

Once again there is no specific treatment for the renal failure. However, colchicine given in a dose of 0·5 mg three times daily is recommended as this therapy appears to abort acute episodes.

Congenital nephrotic syndrome

This term describes the onset of the nephrotic syndrome either 'in utero' or during the first year of life. It may be caused by a variety of conditions including syphilis, toxoplasmosis, mercury poisoning and cytomegalovirus infections. However, the most common cause of the nephrotic syndrome appearing at this time in life is an inherited disorder, particularly common in Finland.

FINNISH TYPE CONGENITAL NEPHROTIC SYNDROME

Inheritance

Transmission is by an autosomal recessive gene.

Pathology

The glomeruli are immature and the capillary tufts small. Many glomeruli are hyalinised and others show mesangial cell proliferation. The cortical tubules are dilated.

Clinical course

The placenta is large, weighing between 25 and 40 per cent of the weight of the infant. Delivery is usually premature and respiratory distress is common. Twenty-five per cent of babies have abdominal distension and oedema at birth and another 25 per cent develop it within the first week. All described cases have developed nephrotic syndrome by the age of three months. The babies have wide cranial sutures and fontanelles, poor somatic development and fail to thrive. Survival beyond the age of two years is rare and infection is the usual cause of death.

Treatment

No effective therapy exists.

DIFFUSE MESANGIAL SCLEROSIS

This is a histological appearance which has been described in a small number of infants who have had a normal placenta and birth weight. Nephrotic syndrome develops shortly after birth and the child dies of uraemia before the age of three. The mode of inheritance is unknown but one pair of identical twins has been affected.

ANOMALIES OF POSITION OF THE KIDNEY
(Fig. 3.1 a, b, c)

Simple renal ectopia

The kidney lies inferior to its normal position, and it fails to rotate so that the ureter joins the anterior surface of the kidney. The renal artery arises from the aorta near the bifurcation or from the common iliac artery. The ureter may drain ectopically.

CLINICAL IMPORTANCE

The condition is usually asymptomatic. The ectopic kidney is more frequently dysplastic than the normally sited kidney. Impaired ureteric drainage may cause stasis and account for recurrent infections which are relatively common.

Crossed renal ectopia

In this position the ectopic kidney lies on the other side of the abdomen and its ureter crosses the midline to drain into the bladder on the normal side. This abnormality is seen once in every 7500 autopsies. The crossed kidney usually lies inferior to the normal kidney and is often fused to its lower pole. The drainage of the

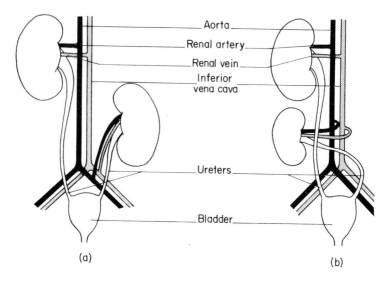

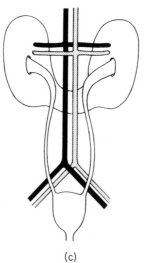

(c)

FIG. 3.1   Anomalous position of the kidney. (a) Simple renal ectopia, (b) crossed renal ectopia, (c) horseshoe kidney.

ectopic kidney may be ectopic or inefficient giving rise to partial obstruction. Carcinomas have occasionally been found in ectopic kidneys.

Renal fusion or horse-shoe kidney

This is found in about 1 in 250 autopsies. The fusion usually occurs between the two lower poles (95 per cent) anterior to the aorta and inferior vena cava. The kidneys are joined by a band of renal parenchyma or fibrous tissue, which prevents the normal rotation of the kidneys. Therefore, the ureters arise anteriorly and run over the isthmus which may cause a degree of obstruction. The clinical consequences stem from this. Horseshoe kidneys are prone to recurrent infection and the formation of calculi. Patients may also suffer episodes of abdominal pain and faintness relieved by leaning forward (Rovsing's syndrome). Both Wilm's tumour and renal cell carcinoma have been reported as arising in these kidneys.

Duplex kidney

Some degree of duplication of the renal pelvis occurs in about 10 per cent of the normal population, but complete duplication giving rise to an extra kidney is remarkably rare.

Clinical consequences of this abnormality are rare, unless the ureters remain separate throughout their length when reflux to the upper moiety is common and may give rise to chronic pyelonephritis. Ectopic opening of one ureter (usually from the upper pole), e.g. into the vagina, may give rise to persistent incontinence.

TREATMENT

If symptoms are present the portion of the kidney drained by the ectopic ureter can be excised surgically.

POINTS OF EMPHASIS

● Many congenital renal abnormalities are of little clinical significance.

- In cases of renal trauma it is wise to know that a contralateral kidney is present before embarking on surgery.

- Unilateral renal hypoplasia may occasionally lead to recurrent infection, stone formation and renal hypertension.

- Bilateral renal hypoplasia is a relatively common cause of terminal renal failure in childhood.

- The incidence of renal dysplasia is increased in ectopic kidneys.

- Most patients with medullary sponge kidneys present between the ages of 20 and 50 with renal colic, haematuria or urinary tract infection. The prognosis is excellent.

- Adult polycystic renal disease is inherited as an autosomal dominant. The clinical course is slowly progressive. The condition accounts for about eight per cent of patients accepted for chronic dialysis in Europe.

- The treatment of polycystic disease largely comprises the management of the complications, which include loin pain, haematuria and renal hypertension, and of progressive renal failure.

- 15 per cent of patients with polycystic renal disease have berry aneurysms of the Circle of Willis.

- The relatives of patients with polycystic disease should be investigated and where appropriate offered genetic counselling once the diagnosis is established.

- Alport's syndrome is the association of progressive nephritis and deafness. It affects males earlier and more severely than females.

- Horseshoe kidneys are prone to infection and stone formation. They may cause abdominal pain and faintness which is relieved by leaning forwards.

- Duplex kidneys may be associated with an increased liability to ureteric reflux into the upper moiety.

- Unexplained retroperitoneal or pelvic masses found at operation may be an ectopic kidney.

CHAPTER 4

Urinary tract infection and interstitial nephritis

INTRODUCTION

Urinary tract infections (UTI) are common. The bladder is more frequently involved than the kidneys. Infections of the upper and lower urinary tract are associated with distinct clinical pictures although both may present with minimal, nondescript symptoms. The relationship between infection and chronic pyelonephritis (which is a common cause of interstitial nephritis) remains unclear.

LOWER URINARY TRACT INFECTION OR CYSTITIS

Clinical course

Increased frequency of micturition, dysuria, urgency, haematuria and lower abdominal pain are common. The symptoms often start abruptly and last for about 7 days even if no treatment is given. Urinary incontinence may be the only indication of infection in the young and elderly and some patients present with vague ill health but no symptoms to point to the urinary tract.

Incidence

A community survey in Wales showed that 22 per cent of women between the age of 20 and 64 had experienced dysuria in the preceding year, and 48 per cent had experienced it at some time. Twelve out of every 1000 visits to general practitioners are caused by the symptoms of 'cystitis'. Cystitis is very rare in males.

Pathogenesis

Only 50 per cent of patients who present to their general practitioner with these symptoms have a positive urine culture. By far the commonest organism is *Escherichia coli* (80–90 per cent). *Bacillus proteus*, *Streptococcus faecalis*, *Staphylococci* and *Pseudomonas* do cause urinary infections but usually in patients with an abnormal urinary tract who have had previous courses of antibiotics or have undergone instrumentation of the urethra. Patients with a negative urine culture have the same symptoms as those with a positive culture but tend to be younger. The term 'urethral syndrome' has been used to describe the association of symptoms with a negative urine culture because it has been suggested that it is an infection of the urethra by organisms spread from the faeces to the introitus and hence to the urethra; the patient then develops symptoms, but a midstream urine remains sterile. There is some evidence to support this hypothesis. Another study has shown that many patients with the urethral syndrome have infections with *Lactobacillus* spp but conventional bacteriological techniques do not reveal these infections because the organism can only be grown in media enriched with carbon dioxide.

Precipitating factors

Sexual intercourse is the commonest factor. It probably causes minor trauma to the urethra and also encourages the retrograde spread of introital organisms into the bladder. Exposure to cold is another factor, although why this should precipitate cystitis is unknown. Bladder catheterisation is the commonest iatrogenic cause of infection. Untreated pelvic sepsis is present in a proportion of patients with recurrent cystitis and adequate treatment of it seems to prevent further attacks of cystitis. Chemical deodorants and vigorous douches are occasionally responsible for recurrent episodes. Lastly, incomplete bladder emptying, which can be detected on the post-micturition film of an intravenous urogram (IVU), may lead to repeated attacks of cystitis.

Diagnosis

The diagnosis of UTI depends on the demonstration of pyuria and a significant number of organisms (greater than 100000/ml urine). A proportion of apparently healthy people are shown to have urinary tract infections when their urine is cultured. These subjects have 'asymptomatic' bacteriuria and numerous epidemiological studies have been performed to identify which group of people with asymptomatic bacteriuria are liable to develop chronic pyelonephritis.

Treatment

An isolated attack may resolve spontaneously. If however the patient presents with symptoms, a course of ampicillin (250 mg six-hourly) or co-trimoxazole (2 tablets twice daily) usually gives relief within 48 hours. The choice of the antibiotic may be influenced by the sensitivity of the infecting organism when this is known. It is not necessary for the course to last longer than five days. A urine culture should be performed about a week after the completion of chemotherapy only if symptoms persist or if the patient is pregnant.

Prevention

Recurrent attacks may be prevented or ameliorated by correcting the precipitating causes if these can be identified. If intercourse is clearly responsible, the patient may benefit from emptying the bladder after intercourse or by taking a tablet of an antibiotic beforehand. Trauma to the introitus may be reduced by applying KY jelly before penetration. All patients benefit from a high fluid intake. Should these measures be insufficient, attacks may be prevented in some patients by taking a tablet of ampicillin, nitrofurantoin or cotrimoxazole every night for a period of six months or more. Dilatation of the urethra has also been widely used by surgeons and does appear to improve symptoms for a few months in some patients. However, it should only be advised if there is evidence of an increased residual urine or a urethral stricture.

'ASYMPTOMATIC' BACTERIURIA

Incidence

This varies with age and sex. In the first year of life more males than females have positive urine cultures and about one per cent of children are affected. Thereafter UTI is very uncommon in males (0·03 per cent) until the seventh decade, when the incidence of infection rises again as prostatic hypertrophy becomes more common. About two per cent of five-year-old girls have infected urine, and five per cent of girls have a UTI at some time during their school career. The incidence in adult women is between three and seven per cent and this appears to be independent of parity and social status. About five per cent of women have a positive urine culture at their first antenatal visit.

Significance

CLINICAL COURSE

The term 'asymptomatic' bacteriuria was poorly chosen because about a third of patients admit to a variety of symptoms such as dysuria, frequency or urgency. Ten per cent have clinical evidence of chronic pyelonephritis. Surveys have also shown that subjects with 'asymptomatic bacteriuria' have a higher blood pressure than people whose urine is sterile. Lastly, pregnant women with bacteriuria on their first antenatal visit have a 30–40 per cent chance of developing acute pyelonephritis during pregnancy.

UNDERLYING STRUCTURAL ABNORMALITIES

Radiological examination of subjects with infected urine reveal renal scars in about ten per cent. The number with ureteric reflux, renal calculi or bladder abnormality varies with the age of the population. Some of these abnormalities may be the effect rather than the cause of the infection.

FOLLOW-UP DATA

Infection tends to resolve spontaneously and to recur periodically. No renal scars have been shown to develop in any group surveyed. This suggests that the development of scars typical of chronic pyelonephritis occurs before the age of five. Renal function (apart from minor defects in concentration) remains excellent despite repeated infections. Therefore, recurrent UTI appears to cause little renal damage providing that no renal scars are present at the age of five, and only has major clinical significance during pregnancy.

TREATMENT

Most patients who have a significant UTI detected are treated, even in the absence of significant symptoms. The therapy described on page 57 is appropriate. However, even if no treatment is given, spontaneous remissions are common. If only half the patients presenting in this way are treated, and an MSU is repeated at the end of one year, there is no significant difference in the incidence of urinary tract infections in the two groups taken at that time.

SCREENING

Routine screening of the urine for infection is only important in patients during pregnancy, in order to prevent the development of acute pyelonephritis, and possibly in hypertensive patients. It should also be undertaken in patients with an abnormal urinary tract, or impaired renal function.

UPPER URINARY TRACT INFECTION

Infections of the renal pelvis or parenchyma may give rise to a well-defined clinical syndrome but the infection may be present in the absence of these symptoms and signs. However, it is doubtful whether exact localisation of a urinary infection to the upper and lower urinary tract is of much clinical importance, and therefore, it is safe to use clinical criteria alone, particularly as some of the techniques for localisation are invasive and potentially hazardous.

Acute pyelonephritis

CLINICAL COURSE

The syndrome varies with age. Young children may present with failure to thrive, vomiting, convulsions or simply a fever. Symptoms referable to the renal tract may be absent. In adults, of whom women are more commonly affected, fever of 39–40°C is common and is associated with loin pain and tenderness which may be very marked. Anorexia and vomiting are also common. Dysuria, frequency and haematuria are often present and the urine may be malodorous.

The natural history of this infection is rarely seen since the diagnosis is usually made and treatment started.

PREDISPOSING CAUSES

Reflux. Vesico-ureteric reflux is common in children: 50 per cent of two-year-olds with UTI have reflux. Infection itself may cause reflux in the young. As the patient grows older reflux becomes less common, and spontaneous cures occur in about 80 per cent of children. Reflux is particularly common in ureters draining kidneys which are scarred.

Obstruction. Any form of obstruction, whether due to congenital anomalies, stones, tumours or prostatic hypertrophy, predisposes to recurrent infection.

Catheterisation. Any catheterisation has about a 5–10 per cent chance of introducing infection, and the incidence of infection rises to almost 100 per cent if the catheter remains *in situ* for four days.

Structural abnormalities of the kidney are also associated with an increased incidence of infection. Polycystic and dysplastic kidneys are good examples.

Diabetes. The incidence of urinary tract infection in diabetes is the same as in the general population, but any infection is usually more severe.

Pregnancy. The incidence of infection is the same as among non-pregnant women, but the chances of developing acute pyelonephritis are much higher. This may be because of the dilatation of the ureter and a degree of urinary stasis which is associated with pregnancy.

DIAGNOSIS

This is made by a positive urine or blood culture in association with a clinical picture and the presence of pyuria. If an IVU is performed during the acute phase, the kidney is enlarged and concentrates the dye less well. During recovery, the kidney returns to normal size. Underlying structural abnormalities particularly those leading to impairment of drainage may be present.

The commonest organism is once again *Escherichia coli*. However, in patients with an uncorrected structural abnormality who have had recurrent courses of antibiotics, other organisms such as *Proteus, Pseudomonas, Enterobacter* and even fungal infections are frequently found.

PATHOLOGY

The kidney is enlarged. Small abscesses develop usually in the medulla but often extending into the cortex. A diffuse interstitial infiltrate with polymorphonuclear leucocytes is found. The pelvic mucosa is grossly congested and the urine contaminated with pus.

TREATMENT

This depends on the severity of the illness. Intravenous fluids may be required for rehydration in which case antibiotics should also be given parenterally. Ampicillin 500 mg six-hourly is a useful choice in a patient presenting for the first time, although another antibiotic may be required if there is no clinical response. By the time that such change is indicated, the results of bacteriological studies of blood and urine should also be available. *Pseudomonas* is common in patients with grossly abnormal renal tracts who have been given several courses of antibiotics. Gentamicin 1–2 mg/kg body weight given 8-hourly or less frequently depending upon renal function or carbenicillin 2 g 6-hourly or cefotaxine 1–3 g 12-hourly are useful in these circumstances. Analgesia should be given to relieve pain. Clinical improvement is usually apparent within two to five days after which it may be possible to finish the course of antibiotic by changing to oral administration if appropriate.

Reflux does not usually require correction in adults. In children, reimplantation of one or both ureters may be required if reflux is so gross as to cause ureteric dilation. The operation is successful in about 80–85 per cent of patients and may dramatically decrease the number of reinfections.

Obstruction should also be sought and corrected. Obviously, no operation should be performed until the acute infection has been controlled.

COMPLICATIONS

Perinephric abscess is a rare but important complication which requires surgical drainage. The diagnosis is made by palpating a mass, or by the demonstration of the mass on IVU or ultrasound examination. Sometimes it is associated with a lack of excretion of dye by the kidney on the affected side.

Septicaemia is not uncommon and may lead to hypotension and metabolic acidosis. Vigorous fluid replacement and parenteral antibiotics are mandatory.

Pyonephrosis is the development of severe infection in an obstructed kidney. The symptoms and signs are the same as for acute pyelonephritis but may be more dramatic. The function of the affected kidney is minimal. Diagnosis may be made by IVU and confirmed by retrograde or antegrade pyelography. Surgical intervention to relieve the obstruction and drain the pus should be performed as soon as the patient's fitness permits.

Papillary necrosis is a rare consequence of renal infection except in a diabetic patient or in a patient with an obstructed kidney.

CHRONIC PYELONEPHRITIS (CPN)

Definition

CPN is the association of a coarse scar in the renal parenchyma with a deformed clubbed calyx underlying it. The diagnosis during life is made by the demonstration of this combination on intravenous urography.

Pathogenesis

The exact age at which these scars develop and the events leading to their formation are still poorly understood. There are several observations which have been used to construct a hypothesis.

1. New scars rarely if ever develop after the age of five unless there is an associated cause, e.g. renal calculi or analgesic abuse.
2. In children, vesico-ureteric reflux is usually demonstrable on the side of the kidney with the scar.
3. Children with reflux are susceptible to recurrent parenchymal infections.

4. Studies in pigs have shown that intrarenal reflux may occur in lobules which drain into a compound papilla, and is unlikely to occur in lobules drained by the more common pyramidal papilla (Fig. 4.1).

5. Intrarenal reflux, either alone or in association with a urinary tract infection, may cause coarse renal scars in pigs.

6. Compound papillae are also found in the human kidney.

7. Organisms are rarely found in the parenchyma of chronic pyelonephritic kidneys.

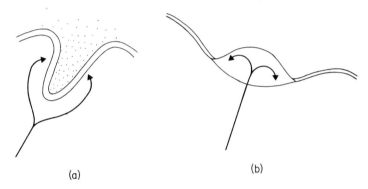

(a)   (b)

FIG. 4.1   (a) Simple papilla. Refluxing urine closes the opening of collecting ducts.
(b) Compound papilla. Refluxing urine opens the orifices of collecting ducts.

Hypothesis

The association of a urinary tract infection with reflux will cause scarring in those lobules of the kidney which drain into compound papillae. This is most likely to happen in the first years of life when reflux is most common. Infection both increases the incidence of reflux and increases the inflammatory response caused by the intrarenal reflux. Healing by fibrosis of the affected lobule leads to both scar formation and associated calyceal distortion.

Pathology

The affected kidney is usually reduced in size although areas of compensatory hypertrophy are often present. Scars may be single or multiple and each is related to a dilated calyx. The distance between the tip of the calyx and the renal capsule may be one-tenth of normal. Scars most commonly form in the polar regions. The contralateral kidney hypertrophies and failure for it to do so may indicate that it also is abnormal.

Histology

The affected area shows both marked tubular loss and a gross interstitial infiltrate consisting of chronic inflammatory cells. The glomeruli are relatively spared, but periglomerular fibrosis is often present. Changes of hypertension may be superimposed. These appearances are not specific to CPN but are seen in many forms of chronic interstitial nephritis.

Incidence

About 20 per cent of patients requiring long-term dialysis in Europe have renal failure due to CPN. Single or multiple scars are found in about ten per cent of subjects with asymptomatic bacteriuria (see above). Post mortem series have given widely differing results, but Heptinstall's series, which is perhaps the most reliable, found changes of CPN in 0·23 per cent with a further 1·41 per cent in whom the changes were associated with urinary tract obstruction.

Clinical

The radiological features of chronic pyelonephritis may be found in a patient who has no symptoms relating to the urinary tract. Recurrent urinary tract infections occur in about 50 per cent of patients with these radiological abnormalities during prolonged follow-up. Common symptoms are low back pain, fever and enuresis as well as dysuria and frequency. Renal tubular abnormalities such as failure to acidify or to concentrate the urine or a failure to conserve sodium are present in many patients but rarely give rise to symptoms. Polyuria and postural hypotension are perhaps the most common symptoms related to tubular dysfunction. Nephrocalcinosis is an occasional radiological finding.

Hypertension may be associated with unilateral or bilateral disease and, especially if untreated, may further aggravate the severity of renal failure. Renal failure is the most serious clinical consequence. Both kidneys must be extensively involved and the progression to renal failure is usually slow, commonly taking between 20 and 40 years. Renal failure may be accelerated by infection or salt depletion, which if corrected can lead to a remarkable degree of recovery of renal function. For more details see Chapter 9. Most patients are either dead or on dialysis by the age of 40.

Treatment

Unfortunately, the exact pathogenesis of scar formation and the age at which it occurs has not yet been defined so it is not possible to prevent the development of the lesions. At present, it seems probable that scars will have formed by the age of five. The relative importance of infection, reflux, shape of papillae and obstruction has yet to be determined.

In children found to have chronic pyelonephritis, long term antibiotic treatment is thought to encourage the growth of the kidneys and, by inference, preserves renal function. In adults, prolonged antibiotic therapy appears to have no influence on the natural history of the disease. However, acute infections should be treated by antibiotics at all ages.

Double micturition should be practiced in all those in whom a residue of dye is seen in the bladder on the post micturition film of the IVU. Obstruction should be sought for, and if found, relieved by surgical correction. Reflux is a more difficult problem, because its exact role has yet to be defined at any particular age. Reflux is more common in the young, and often disappears spontaneously. Therefore, reflux which does not distend the renal pelvis and ureters is probably of little consequence and can be ignored. Severe reflux associated with renal scarring is often taken as an indication for surgical correction which is achieved by re-implanting the ureters into the bladder. The operation is quite successful in preventing reflux (80–85 per cent) but its effect in protecting the kidney from progressive failure is unknown.

Hypertension should be treated by conventional means. The removal of a pyelonephritic kidney may make control of blood pressure much easier, but should only be performed if the other kidney has not been affected by disease. This requires radiological, functional and hormonal studies which should be undertaken by a unit with experience in this problem.

Excessive salt loss may require sodium supplements. Terminal renal failure may be treated by dialysis and transplantation, although bilateral nephrectomy may have to be performed if vesico-ureteric reflux and persistent urinary infections are still present, to prevent the patient's own kidneys becoming an important site for infection when immunosuppressants are being given to inhibit rejection.

URINARY TRACT TUBERCULOSIS

Clinical

The classical presentation of urinary tuberculosis is frequency with sterile pyuria. However, tuberculosis must be considered in the differential diagnosis of almost every urinary tract symptom. The more usual presentations are:

Symptoms of bladder inflammation
    Frequency, dysuria, haematuria
A solitary episode of frank haematuria
Renal colic
Loin pain
Cold abscess in loin
Genital disease
    Male: Epididymitis, orchitis
    Female: Infertility, tubo-ovarian abscess
Chronic renal failure
Routine investigation of:
    Tuberculosis in other organs, including miliary tuberculosis
    Apparently non-tuberculous disease, e.g. hypertension
Constitutional symptoms
Fatigue, anorexia, weight loss

Tuberculosis causes many surgical problems because of the associated fibrosis and ureteric stricture formation.

Diagnosis

It is important to try to prove the diagnosis by obtaining positive culture before treatment is commenced. The following investigations are undertaken to establish the diagnosis and to assess the extent of disease:

Examination of urine
  Bacteriology
  Urinalysis
Radiological examination of the renal tract
Cystoscopy and retrograde pyeloureterography
Estimation of renal function
  Urea and electrolytes
  Creatinine clearance
Radiographic examination of chest
Haematological examination
  Haemoglobin
  Total white blood cells and differential count
  ESR
  Serum folate
Tuberculin test
Examination of genital tract
Identification of previous or concomitant tuberculous disease and of family history of tuberculosis

Treatment

Treatment depends on the extent of urinary tract damage. It is helpful to stage the disease according to the Semb classification 1953 (Fig. 4.2).

Semb I: Tuberculous bacilluria or small calyceal deformity with or without genital lesion
Semb II: Ulcero-cavernous lesion affecting one or more calyces
Semb III: Extensive renal tuberculosis involving the major part of one or more calyces

In general Semb I and II disease can be arrested by antimicrobial therapy, sometimes with the addition of reconstructive surgery because of strictures whereas advanced disease will often necessitate excisional surgery. In recent years, there has been a tendency towards more and more reconstructive surgery, such as the implantation of the ureter into the bladder because of a stricture

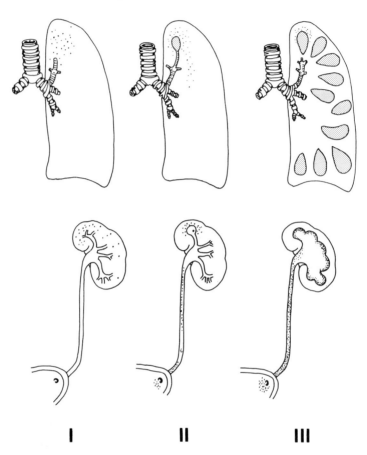

FIG. 4.2 Semb I, II and III classification of renal tuberculosis compared to equivalent pulmonary disease. Redrawn from Semb, Oslo City Hospitals.

at the lower end. Reconstructive surgery is best carried out within the first two months of drug treatment.

The treatment of choice is often six months' chemotherapy with rifampicin and isoniazid, giving pyrazinamide for the initial two months (Table 4.1). Treatment may however have to be adjusted depending upon sensitivities of the infecting organism. In addition, in some developing countries, these expensive anti-tuberculous

TABLE 4.1   Short course chemotherapy for tuberculosis.

Drug	Dosage	Duration
Rifampicin	450 mg	Taken together last thing at night for 2 months
Pyrazinamide	1 g	
Isoniazid	300 mg	
followed by:		
Rifampicin	450 mg	Taken once daily for 7 months.
Isoniazid	300 mg	

Gow, J. G. (1979) Genitourinary tuberculosis: A 7-year review. *British Journal of Urology*, **51**, 239–244.

drugs are not available and it is necessary to use cheaper alternatives and to continue therapy for longer.

Follow-up for longer than one year after the patient has completed treatment is not necessary unless there are doubts about the efficacy of therapy, possibly due to poor patient compliance, or if there are calcified areas on radiology.

SCHISTOSOMIASIS

Schistosomiasis remains one of the commonest causes of haematuria world-wide; it is estimated that five per cent of the world population is infested with one of the forms. The disease, like tuberculosis, causes many problems because of the fibrosis and consequent anatomical distortion. In addition, there is a high incidence of squamous cell carcinoma of the bladder in patients with chronic schistosomal cystitis. This disease should be suspected in anybody with haematuria who has been bathing in fresh water in an endemic area. With the increase of air travel this disease is now seen in holidaymakers as well as immigrants to the UK from endemic areas.

The disease may affect the ureter, bladder, prostate, urethra and external genitalia. The kidneys themselves are rarely directly affected. Effects are inflammation, fibrosis with stricture formation and eventually scarring and calcification. Treatment is with sodium antimony tartrate (a very toxic substance) or niridizole. Drugs should be given for seven days if the infecting organism is *S. haematobium* (Fig. 4.3) and for ten days for *S. mansoni*. Daily dosage regime is 25 mg/kg/day of bodyweight up to a maximum of 1·5 g, best administered in two divided doses. Reconstructive surgery to overcome ureteric stricture is also often necessary.

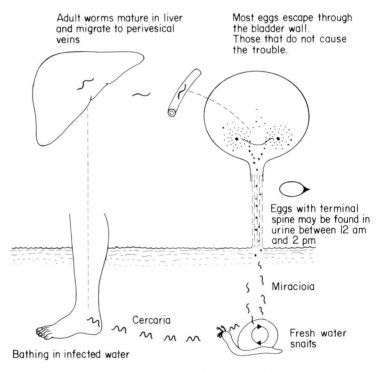

Adult worms mature in liver and migrate to perivesical veins

Most eggs escape through the bladder wall. Those that do not cause the trouble.

Eggs with terminal spine may be found in urine between 12 am and 2 pm

Miracioia

Cercaria

Fresh water snails

Bathing in infected water

FIG. 4.3   The life cycle of *Schistosoma haematobium*.

PAPILLARY NECROSIS

This term describes the process leading to sloughing of one or more papillae. It occurs as a result of analgesic abuse, sickle cell disease, acute pyelitis associated with diabetes or urinary tract obstruction and polyarteritis nodosa. In almost all Western countries, analgesic abuse is by far the commonest cause.

Analgesic nephropathy

This is a capitalist disease. It was first described in small communities in Switzerland and Sweden where the majority were employed in industries liable to cause headaches. It became a habit in these communities to consume large quantities of analgesics prepared by local chemists to their own blend. These analgesics became so popular that they were taken in the same way as chocolates are consumed elsewhere. It was noted that a high proportion of deaths in these small communities were due to renal failure, and in 1953 the link with analgesics was identified. Since then, this association has been confirmed in most areas of the developed world. The incidence is highest in Australia where it is the cause of nearly one-third of patients presenting with renal failure and in the Netherlands where it accounts for about 15 per cent. Elsewhere, it is fortunately less frequent. Each nation has its own favourite brand—Bics in Australia, tabs Codeine Co in England, Askits in Scotland. Phenacetin and aspirin are common to almost all these preparations. Recently, many countries have introduced legislation banning phenacetin from proprietary brands of analgesics but it is still unclear how much this has reduced the incidence of the disease.

Animal experiments have caused some confusion. Vast doses of phenacetin (3000 mg/kg/day for four weeks) are required to cause frank papillary necrosis in rats. It is easier to induce the lesion with aspirin, and this evidence has been used to suggest that phenacetin was not responsible for the disease in man. However, a combination of the two analgesics causes interstitial nephritis and papillary necrosis more easily than either alone. Dehydration accelerates the damage and full hydration appears to protect the animal.

CLINICAL FEATURES

Women are more commonly affected than men. The diagnosis is usually made in the fifth and sixth decade, and relies on an accurate history of analgesic intake.

More than 1 kg of phenacetin has usually been consumed, with an equivalent amount of aspirin. This means that about 4000 tablets or powders have been taken say, six per day for two years. The common reasons for taking this huge amount of analgesics are headaches, rheumatic complaints or simply feeling below par. Not everyone who takes this number of tablets will develop analgesic nephropathy and there may be an inherited factor which predisposes an individual to the disorder.

Early symptoms are very non-specific. Haematuria, urinary tract infection, hypertension, nephrocalcinosis or the finding of sterile pyuria may alert suspicion. Some present with the symptoms of chronic renal failure. The sloughing of a papilla may cause renal colic and/or the passage of fleshy material in the urine. Patients often have symptoms of indigestion and are more anaemic than appropriate for their degree of renal failure. The anaemia is often associated with methaemoglobinaemia and sulphaemoglobin-aemia. Proteinuria is usually less than 1 g/24 hours.

The rate of progression to renal failure depends on the rate of consumption of analgesics.

DIAGNOSIS

This relies on an accurate history and the finding of sterile pyuria. The changes on the IVU depend on the stage of the disease. In the earlier phases, the IVU will be normal and the renal biopsy will show the changes of an interstitial nephritis mainly affecting the medulla. There is an increase in fibrosis and mononuclear cell infiltrate. In the latter stages, the kidney may be reduced in size and pathognomonic changes in the calyces may be found. These are the elongation of the calyceal fornices towards the medulla or the erosion of the base of the papilla which may eventually separate.

Urine assays for para-aminophenol may be helpful in determining whether the patient has recently taken a phenacetin-containing analgesic.

TREATMENT

If the patient can be persuaded to stop taking any analgesic, there is good evidence that some improvement in renal function will occur. However, 50 per cent of patients continue to take analgesics for which there may be a good indication. These patients should be advised to avoid any aspirin, phenacetin or paracetamol preparations and to drink 3–4 litres of liquid per day. There is some animal and clinical evidence that all analgesics (except codeine phosphate) may continue the pathological process. Therefore, patients should be advised to take a single drug such as indomethacin, rather than a composite analgesic and if further deterioration of renal function occurs, they should change again or preferably avoid all analgesics. If terminal renal failure ensues, dialysis and transplantation may be indicated.

CAUSES OF INTERSTITIAL NEPHRITIS

Both pyelonephritis and analgesic nephropathy are causes of an interstitial inflammatory infiltrate but both are also associated with papillary abnormalities and scar formation. The following causes of interstitial nephropathy are usually diffuse and rarely lead to scars or calyceal changes.

Acute interstitial nephritis

AETIOLOGY

Streptococcal and staphylococcal infections may be associated with interstitial oedema and an acute inflammatory exudate. This has recently been described in Legionnaires' disease as well. More commonly drugs are responsible. The penicillins, particularly methicillin, cephalosporins, phenindione, sulphonamides and even frusemide have been reported as causes of an acute interstitial nephritis. A fuller list is given on page 234.

CLINICAL FEATURES

Renal impairment, usually only mild and transient, is associated with fever, rash and often eosinophilia. Occasional patients develop polyuria and failure of acidification may also be present. Substantial or complete recovery of renal function occurs when the infection has been eradicated or the drug withdrawn.

Chronic interstitial nephritis (see Fig. 4.4)

BALKAN NEPHROPATHY

This is a disease affecting people in a narrow area around a 120-mile

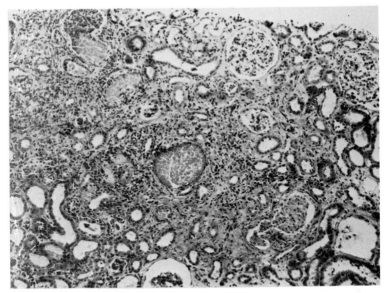

FIG. 4.4 Tubulointerstitial nephritis. There are two normal glomeruli at the top. There is oedema and cellular infiltration in the interstitium with destruction of many tubules. Some tubules are distorted and contain large cellular casts.

length of the river Danube in Yugoslavia and Bulgaria. It accounts for 20 per cent of all deaths in some villages of this area.

Aetiology

This remains unknown. A toxic agent associated with diet or a viral infection have both been postulated.

Clinical features

Symptoms develop after the age of 30 in people born in the area. Immigrants only become ill after living in the area for 10–15 years. Both sexes are equally affected. Dull loin ache, weakness, anorexia and weight loss are the usual presenting symptoms. Haematuria is common, but proteinuria is usually less than 2 g/day. Death occurs within three years and carcinoma of the renal pelvis, ureter or bladder are commonly found.

Treatment

No specific treatment exists.

RADIATION NEPHROPATHY

This may occur if the kidney is exposed to more than 2500 rads, which is now most unusual.

Clinical features

About six months after radiotherapy proteinuria develops and is often massive giving rise to gross oedema. Hypertension and renal failure follow.

Treatment

If only one kidney has been exposed to radiation, nephrectomy may control the hypertension. If however both kidneys have been exposed, control of hypertension is often very difficult by conventional means. Dialysis will be necessary if bilateral nephrectomy is required to control blood pressure.

SJOGREN'S SYNDROME

Only five per cent of patients with Sjogren's syndrome have any abnormality of renal function, and it rarely influences the management of the patient. Occasionally, patients present with progressive renal failure and mild proteinuria. Both kidneys are enlarged, and biopsy reveals a mononuclear interstitial infiltrate. Steroid therapy may be necessary to improve renal function.

GOUT

Gout is associated with an overproduction of uric acid with normal renal handling. Super saturation of the urine with urate leads to:

1. Renal calculi which are found in 15–20 per cent of patients with gout.
2. Massive deposition of urate crystals in tubules leading to obstruction of tubular flow. This is rare and usually found in

patients receiving treatment for myeloproliferative disorders. It causes transient acute renal failure which can be prevented by prior treatment with allopurinol 300 mg daily.

3. Interstitial nephritis caused by an inflammatory reaction to crystals of urate in the tubule and interstitium. Secondary infection and hypertension are common. These changes are commonly found at post mortem, but rarely give rise to progressive renal failure. Treatment with allopurinol can prevent the deposition of further crystals. Hypertension and infection should be controlled.

HEAVY METALS

1. *Lead.* Lead intoxication may give rise to renal insufficiency. Outbreaks have been associated with contamination of wheat and moonshine alcohol and pica in Australia. The more acute features—abdominal colic, anaemia and peripheral neuropathy—dominate the early clinical picture. Insidious renal failure sometimes associated with attacks of gout and hypertension develop later.

2. *Cadmium.* Employees in industries using cadmium have a high incidence of mild renal failure, tubular proteinuria and osteomalacia.

HEREDITARY NEPHRITIS

See Chapter 3.

SARCOIDOSIS

Sarcoid rarely affects the kidneys but an interstitial nephritis associated with progressive renal failure has been described. Steroid therapy is usually effective.

DEPOSITION OF CALCIUM SALTS

Hypercalciuria, hypercalcaemia and oxalosis all lead to deposits of calcium salts in the interstitium and nephrocalcinosis. These will be described in greater detail in Chapter 14. There is some evidence that acceleration of renal failure may occur as the result of interstitial deposits of calcium phosphate crystals in patients with renal failure who have a high product of the serum calcium and phosphate. This may be controlled by adequate intake of phosphate binders thus lowering the serum phosphate.

IDIOPATHIC INTERSTITIAL NEPHRITIS

Some patients present with progressive renal failure, proteinuria of less than 2 g/day and smooth kidneys on IVP. Biopsy material shows minor glomerular abnormalities and a heavy interstitial infiltration with chronic inflammatory cells. No cause can be identified and progression to renal failure is common.

POINTS OF EMPHASIS

● Urinary tract infections are very common.

● The distinction between upper and lower urinary tract infections is not of major clinical importance.

● Only half the women with symptoms of a lower UTI have a positive urine culture using conventional techniques.

● Many lower UTIs resolve spontaneously.

● When attacks can be related to intercourse, their frequency may be reduced by taking an antibiotic before and/or emptying the bladder after sex.

● Recurrent UTIs in adult life are only important in patients with a normal renal tract because of the symptoms they may cause.

● Asymptomatic bacteriuria is of clinical significance in young children and during pregnancy.

● Predisposing factors to acute pyelonephritis include vesico-ureteric reflux, obstruction for any reason, catheterisation, renal structural abnormality and pregnancy.

● Young children with acute pyelonephritis may present with failure to thrive, vomiting, convulsions or fever.

● Suppressive chemotherapy for six months or longer will benefit some patients with recurrent attacks and may prevent renal damage in young children.

- Acute pyelonephritis may be complicated by septicaemia which may progress to bacteraemic shock.

- In the acutely ill patient, parenteral chemotherapy should be initiated as soon as bacteriological samples have been obtained.

- Chronic pyelonephritis (CPN) is a radiological diagnosis comprising the combination of parenchymal scarring with calyceal deformity.

- The link between UTI and CPN remains unclear.

- Scarring usually develops during early childhood and is associated with ureteric reflux, infection, and an abnormal papilla which permits intrarenal reflux.

- Failure of a contralateral kidney to hypertrophy suggests that it also is abnormal.

- 20 per cent of patients requiring long term dialysis have CPN.

- Patients with CPN should be regularly screened for infection and hypertension and, where appropriate, treated for hypertension.

- Analgesic abuse is the commonest cause of papillary necrosis.

- Acute interstitial nephritis may be caused by various infections but is more usually drug-induced.

- Complications of gout can be largely prevented by treatment with allopurinol 300 mg daily.

- Renal tuberculosis may present with almost any urinary symptoms.

- The treatment of choice in renal tuberculosis is usually six months' therapy with rifampicin and isoniazid giving pyrazinamide in addition for the initial two months during which any reconstructive surgery is best performed.

CHAPTER 5

Tubular dysfunction and electrolyte abnormalities

Normal renal tubular function is essential to the maintenance of the constancy of the volume of body fluids, as well as their pH and salt composition. This chapter surveys some of the commoner tubular abnormalities which have consequences of clinical importance and describes some of the causes of electrolyte disturbances. However, clinically significant disturbances of tubular function are all rare.

ABNORMALITIES OF pH

Acidosis (see Fig. 1.11)

Normal people generate about 1 mmol/kg/day of H^+. The proximal renal tubular cells respond to systemic acidosis by generating more bicarbonate which is transferred to the blood. For each molecule of bicarbonate generated, 1 molecule of H^+ is excreted as water (Fig. 1.10). This is a continuous process which takes a few days to fully develop. The second renal response is to increase the secretion of H^+ by the distal tubular cell. Secreted hydrogen ions are buffered by ammonia, phosphates and other systems.

Failure of either of these two systems may lead to a metabolic acidosis even when production of H^+ is not increased.

Acidosis of renal failure

This may occur in progressive renal failure whatever the cause. The plasma bicarbonate concentration falls but there is no commensurate rise in the chloride level. Thus the anion gap is increased (i.e. $Na - (Cl + HCO_3)$ is usually less than 12). The 'missing' anions are phosphate, sulphate and other organic acids retained in renal failure.

Renal tubular acidosis (RTA)

Failure of the tubular function of acidification results in the formation of an inappropriately alkaline urine in a patient with systemic acidosis. The severity of the disorder varies, and some patients have a normal plasma pH under basal conditions but are unable to acidify the urine when given an acid load and thus develop a systemic acidosis.

Definition

Any patient with systemic acidosis, indicated by a reduced plasma bicarbonate, whose urinary pH is above 5·4 *or* any patient in whom the urinary pH does not fall below 5·4 within six hours of being given ammonium chloride 0·1 g/kg orally.

CLASSIC, TYPE I OR DISTAL RENAL TUBULAR ACIDOSIS

In this disorder, there is a failure of the distal tubular cell to secrete H^+. This leads to an increased loss of sodium and potassium ions. Nephrocalcinosis, stone formation and rickets or osteomalacia develop as a result of hypercalciuria. If uncorrected, progressive reduction in glomerular filtration rate may occur.

Causes

Familial. Transmission is by an autosomal dominant gene.

Acquired. Distal RTA occurs as part of many other renal diseases which mainly affect the medulla, e.g. pyelonephritis or hydronephrosis. Any condition producing hypercalciuria is also commonly associated with this type of RTA e.g. hypervitaminosis D or medullary sponge kidney. Hypergammaglobulinaemia is another association. This may be a part of Sjogren's syndrome or a multi-system auto immune disease of which the other components may be chronic active hepatitis, fibrosing alveolitis and peripheral neuropathy.

Clinical features

Muscle weakness, growth retardation and rickets are common in children. Osteomalacia develops in adults. Polyuria and polydipsia result from a failure of urinary concentration. Constipation is common. X-ray of the abdomen may reveal extensive nephrocalcinosis.

The plasma concentration of potassium and bicarbonate are reduced and chloride raised. The urinary pH is above 5·4 but rarely contains bicarbonate. Some patients with an incomplete form may have a normal plasma bicarbonate but fail to acidify the urine in response to an ammonium chloride load as described above.

Treatment

Correction of acidosis by oral sodium and potassium citrate (Shohl's solution) may improve all abnormalities and prevent further decline in renal function unless gross nephrocalcinosis is already present when the diagnosis is made. Between 5 and 12 mmol of alkali per kg body weight per day is usually required. Gross osteomalacia or rickets may heal with alkalis alone, but healing will be accelerated by giving 1 α-hydroxycholecalciferol 0·25–1·0 μg per day.

TYPE II OR PROXIMAL RENAL TUBULAR ACIDOSIS

Lesions of the proximal convoluted tubule may result in the failure of reabsorption of filtered bicarbonate. Since distal tubular function remains intact, low urinary pH (below 5·4) may be achieved when the filtered bicarbonate is drastically reduced, as happens in severe metabolic acidosis. Hypokalaemia and nephrocalcinosis do not occur, thus distinguishing the clinical presentation from that of Type I RTA.

Causes

1. Carbonic anhydrase deficiency. This enzyme is in the brush border of the proximal tubule cell and is responsible for the acceleration in the reabsorption of bicarbonate (see Fig. 1.10).

Carbonic anhydrase may be absent as an inherited disorder or as a result of treatment with acetazolamide.

2. In association with diseases of the proximal tubule as occur in Wilson's disease and Lowe's syndrome. Hypocalcaemia and secondary hyperparathyroidism, myeloma and out-dated tetracycline may also cause proximal renal tubular acidosis.

Clinical features

The clinical features of proximal tubular acidosis are much less severe than distal tubular acidosis and the other clinical manifestations of the associated condition usually dominate the clinical picture.

Treatment

Treatment is by giving alkali. Chlorothiazide may reduce the amount of alkali required and is an adjunct to therapy.

Alkalosis

The kidney usually plays only a secondary role in most of the causes of metabolic alkalosis.

Vomiting. Prolonged and severe vomiting may lead to a loss of H^+ so great, that were the kidney to waste the equivalent amount of bicarbonate to maintain the pH, sodium depletion and accelerated circulatory collapse would result. Therefore potassium is excreted in preference to H^+ ions by the kidney. For this reason persistent vomiting results in considerable hypokalaemic alkalosis.

Drugs. Steroids, diuretics, liquorice derivatives and purgatives in excessive quantities all cause hypokalaemic alkalkosis.

Mineralocorticoid overproduction. This occurs in various relatively rare syndromes such as renal artery stenosis, malignant hypertension, Conn's and Cushing's syndromes, and the overproduction of deoxycorticosterone. Mineralocorticoids cause an increased sodium reabsorption in the distal tubule leading to an equivalent increment in the secretion of potassium and H^+ thus causing hypokalaemic alkalosis. As the hypokalaemia develops H^+

ions enter cells in exchange for K^+ ions thereby aggravating the alkalosis. However, increase in extracellular sodium leads to expansion of extracellular volume by 2–3 litres and thereafter there is an increase in filtered sodium and bicarbonate which limits the alkalosis, as bicarbonate reabsorption is incomplete and some is lost in the urine.

Milk-alkali syndrome. The ingestion of alkali rarely leads to systemic alkalosis because the kidney is very efficient at excreting an alkaline load. If however, the alkali is taken with a sufficient quantity of calcium, e.g. as in milk, to cause hypercalcaemia and nephrocalcinosis, then alkalosis may develop, particularly if the patient loses acid by vomiting. This often happens, since peptic ulceration is the usual cause for the ingestion of the combination of milk and alkali. Hypercalcaemia, hyperphosphataemia and hypoparathyroidism all decrease the ability of the kidney to excrete an alkaline load. This syndrome is rare.

Bartter's syndrome. This is another rare syndrome and will be described on page 93.

ABNORMALITIES OF CONCENTRATION

Failure of concentration

The development of an efficient mechanism to concentrate urine was an essential prerequisite to life on land. Animals living in deserts have an extraordinary power of concentration; the chinchilla, for example, can raise its urine osmolarity to 7500 mosmol/kg. In man, the range is more modest, but osmolarities between 50 and 1400 mosmol/kg can be achieved. Failure to concentrate the urine results in polyuria of between 5 and 10 litres/day. There are many causes.

VASOPRESSIN-SENSITIVE DIABETES INSIPIDUS

This is caused by a failure of production of antidiuretic hormone (ADH) by the hypothalamus.

Aetiology

Hypophysectomy is now the commonest cause. Tumours and hypothalamic trauma may also result in diabetes insipidus. The condition may be inherited as an autosomal dominant or be found without obvious cause.

Clinical features

Severe thirst and polyuria are the most obvious symptoms. The patient is usually slightly dehydrated and serum osmolarity slightly raised (285–300 mosmol/kg). The urine osmolarity is usually less than that of the serum. The bladder may be huge, and the ureters and calyces dilated, as in any form of severe sustained diuresis. Periods of unconsciousness are particularly hazardous, as fluid replacement may stop and the patient becomes grossly dehydrated.

Investigations

The first step is to carefully measure 24-hour urinary volumes over several days to test the accuracy of the patient's history. Urine volumes of less than three litres while the patient is allowed to drink normally are unlikely to be associated with significant disease. If, however, urine volumes are considerably in excess of this, the patient should be admitted for a water deprivation test. This must be performed under close supervision, to ensure that the patient does not become dangerously dehydrated. The patient should be weighed accurately and then deprived of water until there has been a reduction of three per cent in body weight. The urine osmolarity should rise above 800 mosmol/kg. If the urinary osmolarity remains less than this, aqueous pitressin (5 units) should be infused intravenously over one hour. There should be a prompt increase in urine osmolarity in patients with diabetes insipidus, but in patients with nephrogenic diabetes insipidus (see below) there is no such increase.

Treatment

Vasopressin tannate in oil 2–5 units every two to three days is effective, but reactions occur in some patients. Desmopressin (dDAVP) is a new synthetic preparation which can be taken intranasally; 20 mg is effective for 24 hours and this is now the treatment of choice. In patients who have some residual ADH secretion, oral therapy with chlorpropramide, clofibrate or carbamazepine may be helpful.

NEPHROGENIC DIABETES INSIPIDUS (NDI)

Aetiology

This syndrome has many causes. It is frequently found in patients with chronic renal failure caused by disease processes affecting the medulla, e.g. obstructive uropathy, hypercalcaemia or medullary cystic disease. It is also a feature of hypokalaemia. Some drugs such as methoxyflurane, lithium and demeclocycline have also been reported to cause transient polyuria. Lastly, nephrogenic diabetes insipidus may be inherited as a sex-linked recessive.

Clinical features

The extent of the polyuria varies from patient to patient, but very large urinary volumes are unusual in patients with chronic renal failure. Unlike vasopressin-responsive diabetes insipidus, NDI is often associated with large losses of urinary sodium. Very large urinary losses of water and electrolytes may follow the relief of obstructive uropathy. The clinical presentation of inherited nephrogenic diabetes insipidus is very similar to that of vasopressin-sensitive diabetes insipidus.

Treatment

Early diagnosis is essential in the inherited form to prevent severe dehydration and brain damage. Adequate fluid replacement remains the cornerstone of management. Chlorothiazide and other diuretics reduce urine volume and are helpful.

POLYURIA DUE TO SOLUTE LOAD

Alcohol intake is perhaps the most natural example of diuresis induced by solute. However, the most important clinical example is diabetes mellitus. An increase in extracellular glucose leads to intracellular dehydration as water leaves the cell along the osmotic gradient. Water is excreted in increased amounts as a direct result of the expanded extracellular volume and more importantly because of the osmotic load of glucose in the urine. Extracellular fluid depletion results. The diuretic action of osmotic diuretics is based on the same principle. As already mentioned, patients with a salt losing nephropathy also lose large volumes of water in the urine.

Failure of dilution

INAPPROPRIATE SECRETION OF ANTIDIURETIC HORMONE (SIADH)

If ADH is given to a healthy subject for several days, the urine volume initially will fall and body weight will rise as water is reabsorbed. Sodium excretion gradually rises in response to the expanded extracellular volume and so the plasma sodium concentration and plasma osmolarity fall. The urine osmolarity rises initially, but falls slowly over the next few days as a new steady state develops. These changes can be reversed by reducing water intake.

Aetiology

These changes may occur in patients with:

1. Pulmonary infections of any cause. Hyponatraemia is usually mild and reverts to normal when the infection is cured, but can be severe in advanced pulmonary tuberculosis.
2. Various tumours, particularly bronchogenic carcinomas. This is the second most common cause of SIADH. ADH is produced ectopically in the tumour, and hyponatraemia will persist unless all the secreting tumour is removed (see below).
3. Lesions of the central nervous system. Head injury, subarachnoid haemorrhage, meningitis, encephalitis and brain tumours have all been associated with SIADH.
4. Stress such as pain, anxiety or surgery, which may lead to hyponatraemia due to increased production of ADH by the neurohypophysis.
5. Drugs. Vasopressin and oxytocin overdose can, of course, produce the syndrome. Chlorpropamide increases the sensitivity of the renal tubule to ADH and may cause dilutional

hyponatraemia. Vincristin, cyclophosphamide, clofibrate and carbamazepine have also been implicated.

Clinical features

A mild increase in body water may be symptomless but it may cause heart failure in patients with cardiac disease. More severe dilution, causing a serum sodium of 105–110 mmol/l, may be associated with confusion, drowsiness, coma or convulsions.

Investigations

The following are characteristics of the syndrome:

1. Low serum sodium and osmolarity.
2. Inappropriately high urine osmolarity. This is usually higher than the osmolarity of the serum but in the chronic phase, the urine osmolarity may be less than that of serum.
3. Raised ADH concentration.
4. The urine sodium will reflect sodium intake, and is usually relatively high.

Causes of impaired tubular function such as the taking of diuretics or analgesics should be excluded.

Treatment

The underlying cause should be sought and treated appropriately.

Acute. Hypertonic (2N) saline may be given to the comatose patient. A diuretic may be required in patients with cardiac decompensation because extracellular fluid volume would be increased further.

Subacute. Water intake should be reduced to 500 ml/day and the serum sodium and body weight monitored. When the serum sodium has returned to within the normal range, the weight of the patient should be noted and fluid intake adjusted to keep it at that level.

Chronic. Demeclocycline 300 mg 12-hourly increases free water clearance and has few side effects. It is effective in ameliorating the symptoms in most patients in whom the underlying disorder cannot be treated.

DISORDERS OF TRANSPORT

There are many disorders of tubular transport, most of which are rare and of little clinical significance. The following account is highly selective. Proximal tubular disorders are associated with failure of transport of glucose, phosphate and certain amino acids.

Cystinuria

This is a disorder of defective transport of cystine, ornithine, arginine and lysine. Increased amounts of these amino acids are excreted in the urine. The disorder is of clinical importance because of the low solubility of cystine in the urine.

Inheritance

This is as an autosomal recessive, although heterozygotes excrete increased amounts of lysine and cystine.

Clinical features

Cystine stones form in the urinary tract causing renal colic, haematuria and recurrent infection. The stones are moderately radio-opaque.

Diagnosis

Increased excretion of the four amino acids can be found in the urine. Flat hexagonal crystals of cystine may be seen on urinary microscopy.

Treatment

Surgical removal of stones may be necessary. The prevention of new stone formation may be achieved by either increasing fluid intake to five litres per day and alkalising the urine with sodium bicarbonate or by the chronic administration of penicillamine 1–3 g/day.

The Lignac–Fanconi syndrome

IN CHILDREN

This is a disorder caused by the absence of an enzyme, cystine reductase. Deposits of cystine are laid down all over the body and may be identified in the cornea or white cells. There is a swan neck deformity of the proximal tubule. The tubular abnormality leads to a loss of phosphate, urate, glucose and amino acids in the urine and renal tubular acidosis (Type II).

Inheritance

Transmission is by an autosomal recessive gene.

Clinical features

Children present within a few months of birth with failure to thrive, vomiting, polyuria, polydipsia and rickets.

Investigations

Hypokalaemia, acidosis, low serum urate and hypophosphataemia are found in association with increased losses of urate, glucose and amino acids in the urine.

Treatment

Rickets should be treated by 1 α-hydroxycholecalciferol (1α-OHCC); the electrolyte and pH upset is corrected by Shohl's solution and a high fluid intake should be encouraged.

Prognosis

Death usually occurs within a few months.

IN ADULTS

This is a rare disorder, secondary to a variety of conditions such as Wilson's disease or fructose intolerance. The combination of glycosuria with a normal blood sugar, aminoaciduria, phosphaturia, hypokalaemia and low serum urate is typical. Systemic acidosis may also be present. The patient usually presents with osteomalacia.

Treatment

1 α-OHCC and Shohl's solution correct most of the abnormalities, but slow deterioration of renal function is usual.

Lowe's syndrome (oculocerebrorenal dystrophy)

This is another rare disorder.

Inheritance

Sex linked recessive.

Clinical features

Infants present at birth with cataracts, buphthalmos causing blindness of varying degree, muscular hypotonia and mental retardation. Renal glycosuria, acidosis, aminoaciduria and hypophosphataemia are found.

Prognosis

Death usually occurs within a few years from renal failure or from infection.

Vitamin D resistant rickets

Inheritance

There are two varieties. One is inherited as a sex linked dominant and the other is an autosomal recessive. The former type is due to decreased phosphate reabsorption and the latter is associated with a deficiency of the enzyme l-hydroxylase which leads to decreased production of 1,25-dihydroxycholecalciferol.

Clinical presentation

Both forms present as rickets in childhood.

Treatment

Treatment is by 1 α-OHCC in physiological doses.

DISORDERS OF ELECTROLYTES

Hyponatraemia

Hyponatraemia may be due to sodium depletion or water retention or a combination of both. Patients with hyponatraemia may be subdivided according to the clinical estimate of the extracellular volume.

Hyponatraemia associated with a high extracellular fluid volume is seen in:

1. Congestive cardiac failure, hepatic failure or the nephrotic syndrome treated by diuretics and restricted sodium intake, but with no restriction of the water intake *or* when potassium replacement is inadequate.

2. Syndrome of inappropriate ADH secretion (see above).

3. Polydipsia. If the amount of water drunk exceeds the capacity of the kidney to excrete it, hyponatraemia results. Primary polydipsia is extremely rare.

4. Myxoedema. The reason for hyponatraemia in this condition is unknown.

Hyponatraemia associated with normal extracellular fluid volume is seen in:

1. Patients in (1) above but in whom diuretics have removed excess extracellular fluid.

2. 'False hyponatraemia'. An apparently low serum sodium concentration may occur in patients with very high plasma lipid or protein concentrations. The volume taken by these molecules is included in the volume used to calculate the concentration of sodium whereas the true aqueous volume is less; therefore, an inappropriately low concentration of sodium results.

3. Postoperative. When fluid volume replacement is correct but only 5 per cent dextrose is used.

Hyponatraemia associated with a reduced extracellular volume is seen in:

1. Hypovolaemia. Most patients with a degree of hypovolaemia will have a moderately reduced plasma sodium concentration.
2. Addison's disease. Because of the therapeutic implications, this possibility should be excluded whenever there is any doubt.
3. Sick cell syndrome.

Treatment

The treatment is essentially that of the underlying cause. In patients with increased extracellular volume, water intake should be restricted. In those with severely depleted extracellular volume, e.g. in Addisonian crisis, hypertonic saline may be required. The hyponatraemia of severe congestive cardiac failure is often resistant to treatment but removal of fluid by ultrafiltration across a dialysis membrane may lead to a satisfying if temporary improvement.

Hypernatraemia

Severe hypernatraemia is rare and is seen in patients presenting with:

1. Diabetic decompensation, particularly hyperosmolar non-ketotic diabetic coma.
2. Malignancy.
3. Expanded extracellular fluid volume.

Hypokalaemia

Hypokalaemia is usually associated with alkalosis. Its presence indicates a substantial deficit of total body potassium and is always due to abnormal losses by the kidney, the alimentary tract, or both. Urinary potassium losses will be disproportionate to the degree of hypokalaemia if the primary problem is renal.

Primary renal causes

1. Drugs which include all diuretics (except those acting on the distal tubule), steroids and carbenoxolone.

2. Endogenous overproduction of mineralcorticosteroids such as occurs in Conn's and Cushing's syndromes, renal artery stenosis or malignant hypertension.

3. Diabetic ketoacidosis. Severe potassium depletion may occur as a result of the osmotic diuresis and may be aggravated by vomiting, but the patient may be hyperkalaemic initially. This depletion will become unmasked during insulin therapy, especially if bicarbonate is given to correct the acidosis.

4. Bartter's syndrome. This is a rare disease of early childhood. The child fails to thrive and has polyuria, hypokalaemia and an increased loss of potassium in the urine. He is usually normotensive despite elevated levels of renin, angiotensin, aldosterone. The renal biopsy appearances are abnormal only in that the juxtaglomerular apparatus is hypertrophied. The cause of the syndrome is unknown but some patients are helped by a prostaglandin inhibitor e.g. indomethacin 25 mg tds.

5. Hypokalaemia may also occur in association with renal tubular acidosis.

Primary alimentary causes

1. Vomiting, if prolonged (see page 82).
2. Severe diarrhoea, including self-abuse of purgatives.

FEATURES

Tiredness and lethargy are common features which may progress to muscle weakness and even paralysis. There is increased myocardial excitability and dangerous arrhythmias may occur, particularly in the elderly or in patients taking digoxin.

MANAGEMENT

Mild degrees of hypokalaemia are best treated with oral supplements, preferably by a slow release preparation such as Slow-K 0·6–3·6 g day (8–48 mmol/day). Severe losses of potassium should be replaced intravenously. In diabetic ketoacidosis massive doses of potassium may be required, but it is unwise to exceed 1·5 g/h (20 mmol/h). Regular measurements of serum K^+ should be made.

Hyperkalaemia

Hyperkalaemia may result from a failure to excrete potassium, as occurs in renal failure. This is of especial clinical importance in acute renal failure (see Chapter 8). It may also occur in states of metabolic acidosis when H^+ is moved intracellularly in exchange for potassium in order to minimise the acidosis. Excess potassium is excreted in the urine and therefore hyperkalaemia can be associated with a reduced total body potassium (as in diabetes—see above).

POINTS OF EMPHASIS

● Clinically significant disturbances of tubular function are rare.

● Distal RTA, unlike proximal RTA, is often associated with nephrocalcinosis and untreated may cause progressive renal failure.

● Persistent vomiting results in severe hypokalaemic alkalosis.

● Failure of urinary concentration occurs in vasopressin-sensitive and nephrogenic diabetes insipidus and when there is an excessive solute load.

● In untreated vasopressin-sensitive diabetes insipidus, urinary osmolarity is usually less than that of the serum.

● Unlike vasopressin-sensitive diabetes insipidus, nephrogenic diabetes insipidus is often associated with large losses of urinary sodium.

● A mild increase in body water may cause heart failure in patients with cardiac disease.

● Cystine stone formation can be prevented either by high fluid and alkaline intake or by penicillamine.

● Hyponatraemia may occur with a high, low or normal extracellular fluid volume.

● Addison's disease is a rare but a therapeutically important cause of hyponatraemia.

● Significant hypokalaemia is always due to abnormal potassium losses either via the kidney or the alimentary tract.

CHAPTER 6

Primary glomerulopathies

INTRODUCTION

Almost all forms of glomerular injury are the result of systemic disorders which lead to renal damage. In many patients, the nature of the systemic disorder has not been discovered and the only event of clinical importance is the injury to the glomeruli; this group makes up the primary glomerulopathies. Attempts to classify them clinically have been unsuccessful so the introduction of the technique of percutaneous renal biopsy in 1951 was quickly developed and led to a detailed pathological classification, which is now generally accepted.

The entities described are not diseases in themselves. This became apparent when immunofluorescent studies of renal biopsies showed that one pathogenetic mechanism was capable of causing more than one pathological lesion. However, a pathogenetic classification of the glomerulopathies has not been achieved as yet. The ideal classification would be one which identified the aetiological agent responsible for triggering off the mechanism causing glomerular injury. Unfortunately, the causes of the great majority of glomerulopathies remain unknown, and the pathological classification is still used because it remains the best available. Table 6.1 shows the four levels of classification.

TABLE 6.1

Clinical
Persistent proteinuria
Nephrotic syndrome
Acute nephritic syndrome
Hypertension
Chronic renal failure
Recurrent haematuria

Pathological
Minimal change nephropathy
Focal glomerulosclerosis
Membranous nephropathy
The proliferative nephropathies

Pathogenetic
Anti-GBM nephritis
Immune complex nephritis
Unknown

Aetiological
Infections
Tumours
Drugs
Autoantibodies

CLINICAL PRESENTATION OF THE GLOMERULOPATHIES

There are only a limited number of clinical consequences of glomerular damage.

Persistent proteinuria

Normal subjects lose up to 150 mg of protein in their urine each day, of which about 10 mg is albumin and the rest is of tubular origin such as the Tam Horsfall protein and $\beta2$ microglobulin. The amount of protein in the urine may be increased on standing. In some individuals, the change in posture may lead to quite large losses of protein. This is called orthostatic proteinuria. Most patients with this disorder have no serious glomerular abnormality but this is not always so; the fact that urine is free of protein when the patient is lying down should not contraindicate investigation by renal biopsy. Mild proteinuria causes no symptoms except perhaps an unusual frothiness of the urine and it is usually discovered at routine medical examinations.

Nephrotic syndrome

PATHOPHYSIOLOGY

Urinary loss of protein leads to increased albumin synthesis by the liver. If the loss is large, or if the patient has inadequate dietary intake of nitrogen or calories, then the increase in albumin synthesis is insufficient to replace urinary loss and hypoalbuminaemia results. This in turn decreases the oncotic pressure of blood and leads directly to oedema formation. Proteinuria, hypoalbuminaemia and oedema are the hallmarks of the nephrotic syndrome. Hypercholesterolaemia is usually present, although the reason for this is not understood.

The transfer of fluid from the circulation to the extracellular space decreases the circulating volume. This promotes retention of salt and water by increased secretion of aldosterone and antidiuretic hormone, thus restoring the circulating volume and increasing the oedema. Swelling is the main complaint of patients but it also, in part, represents the body's attempt to correct the loss of circulating volume. Therefore, over-vigorous attempts to remove the oedema may reduce circulating volume and decrease renal flow and renal function.

CLINICAL FEATURES

Oedema is the most obvious and troublesome symptom. Children tend to have facial oedema and ascites while adults have ankle and leg oedema when standing and sacral and facial oedema when lying. Very low serum albumin often gives rise to anorexia, nausea and vomiting. The nephrotic syndrome is associated with an increased liability to infections and to accelerated atheroma formation due to the common associations with hypertension, hyperlipidaemia and hypercoagulable state. Myocardial infarction is thought to occur more commonly and at a younger age in nephrotics than in the normal population, although this has recently been challenged.

TREATMENT

Most patients with nephrotic syndrome present with oedema. The following measures may reduce the swelling, when renal function is well preserved.

Protein in diet. The maximum plasma albumin concentration for any degree of proteinuria may be achieved by ensuring an adequate protein and calorie intake. Very high protein diets are expensive and nauseating and have no proven advantage over protein intake of 1·5 g/kg/day in adults. Children may require considerably more. more.

Diuretics. The increase in extracellular fluid may be reduced by giving oral diuretics to promote loss of salt and water. The dose of diuretic should be titrated against the patient's weight, and renal function should be carefully monitored as reduction in circulating volume may lead to a reduction in renal function.

   1. *Bendrofluazide* 5 to 10 mg/day is a mild, cheap and long-acting diuretic which may be sufficient for minimal oedema and is particularly useful if the patient is also hypertensive.
   2. *Frusemide* is the most commonly used diuretic. It is potent and short acting. Therefore, frusemide 40 mg every morning may cause a brisk diuresis which wears off by midday, so that oedema tends to reaccumulate towards evening. For this reason, it is better to give a second tablet (of 40 mg) at noon rather than to increase the morning dose. The severity of the diuresis may make it impractical for a working person if their job is away from easy access to a lavatory. The dose of frusemide may be progressively increased until a dose of 500 mg twice daily is reached. Frusemide is available as 20 mg, 40 mg, and 500 mg tablets and for injection in ampoules of 20 mg, 50 mg, and 250 mg.
   3. The thiazide diuretics act on the proximal tubules, frusemide on the loop of Henle. Therefore, a diuretic which acts on the distal tubules is a useful adjunct. *Spironolactone* (an aldosterone antagonist) is a good example. It is a mild diuretic and encourages the reabsorption of potassium, which is wasted by the diuretics whose action is more proximal. It may be given in doses ranging from 25 mg per day to 100 mg four times a day.

Salt and water restriction. Some patients with gross oedema are apparently resistant to even the severest diuretic regime, usually because they replenish their extracellular volume of fluid by drinking more. These patients should be asked to reduce their 24 hour intake to about one litre and to restrict their salt intake to 40 mmol/24 h. The effect of treatment should be measured by weighing the patient daily (if in hospital) or at each visit to the out-patient clinic.

Some patients with massive proteinuria are both oedematous and ill, suffering from anorexia, nausea, vomiting and loss of muscle mass. These patients should be admitted to hospital and given salt-poor albumin intravenously to restore circulating volume. As much as 100 g albumin may have to be given daily for a few days. It is very expensive and the beneficial effect may only last a few days as urinary loss is rapid. Diuretics should be given at the same time so that the extracellular fluid volume is rapidly reduced, while the circulating volume is maintained by intravenous albumin. This regime is useful in tiding a patient over a crisis, and may have to be repeated from time to time in the occasional patient who has persistent massive proteinuria.

Indomethacin has been used to reduce proteinuria but a controlled trial showed that its effect was temporary, there being no difference in the proteinuria of the control and treated groups at six months. However, it may be useful in a rare individual.

The nephritic syndrome

PATHOPHYSIOLOGY

The nephritic syndrome differs from the nephrotic syndrome in that there is expansion of both the circulating and extracellular fluid volumes. The cause of fluid retention is not fully understood. Patients usually continue to take a normal fluid intake (until advised not to), and if oliguria is present, this leads to accumulation of fluid. The second contributory factor is an inappropriately high tubular reabsorption of sodium. Whatever the precise mechanism, salt and water retention is responsible for the major clinical findings of patients with the nephritic syndrome.

CLINICAL FEATURES

The first symptom of the acute nephritic syndrome is usually a reduction in urine volume. The urine may be smoky or frankly blood stained. The patient then becomes oedematous which may first be noticed as a peri-orbital puffiness. On examination, the signs of expansion of the circulatory volume are found—tachycardia, raised blood pressure, raised jugular venous pressure, a gallop rhythm and sometimes crepitations at the lung bases. Facial and ankle oedema are usual.

INVESTIGATIONS

A variable degree of renal failure may be found. The serum albumin is usually only moderately reduced. The urine contains protein, red cells and red cell casts. A raised ASOT and a low serum C3 are found in the majority of patients, as described under acute exudative glomerulonephritis (see below). Renal biopsy is indicated unless there is clear evidence of a streptococcal aetiology in which case it should only be performed if the natural history is unusual (see below).

TREATMENT

If renal failure is present, this should be managed as outlined in Chapter 9. It is sometimes possible to provoke a diuresis with large doses of frusemide. Salt, water, potassium and protein intake should be restricted and the blood pressure controlled by conventional means.

ASSOCIATIONS

The acute nephritic syndrome is associated with acute exudative glomerulonephritis, which usually follows a streptococcal infection. It is more rarely seen in patients with mesangiocapillary or rapidly progressive glomerulonephritis. Very occasionally patients with mesangial IgA disease have a mild form of the syndrome.

Hypertension

This is common in a varying proportion of patients with all forms of glomerulopathy and may be the presenting complaint. It should be treated as outlined on pages 194–6.

Chronic renal failure

Many patients with progressive glomerulopathy present with consequences of the insidious development of chronic renal failure (see Chapter 9).

Recurrent haematuria

Episodes of frank haematuria usually following upper respiratory tract infections are a rarer presentation of glomerulopathy and occur most often in young men between the ages of 15 and 25. Haematuria may also be provoked by exercise.

ASSOCIATIONS

Mesangial IgA (Berger's) disease is the most common form of glomerulopathy associated with this presentation. Rarely patients with mesangiocapillary glomerulonephritis may present in this way.

PATHOLOGICAL CLASSIFICATION OF GLOMERULOPATHIES

The indications for performing a renal biopsy are described on page 37.

Minimal change nephropathy (MCN) (Lipoid nephrosis or idiopathic nephrotic syndrome)

PATHOLOGY

Light microscopy (LM)

Glomeruli and tubules appear normal in most instances. There may be a slight increase in the mesangial matrix or mesangial cell numbers (Fig. 6.1).

Electron microscopy (EM)

The only constant abnormality is one of epithelial foot process fusion. No electron dense deposits are found.

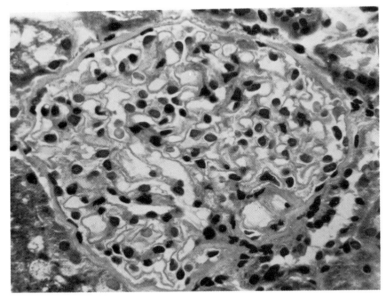

FIG. 6.1   Normal glomerulus.

Immunofluorescent studies (IF)

No deposits of immunoglobulins or complement components are found in the majority of biopsies. Small deposits of IgM and C3 both within the glomeruli and around the afferent arterioles are sometimes seen. Their significance is unknown.

CLINICAL FEATURES

Age

The peak incidence of presentation of this syndrome is between the ages of 2 and 5. It is the cause of the nephrotic syndrome in 90 per cent of children and 25 per cent of adults.

Sex

In childhood, two boys are affected for every girl, but in adults there is no sex preference.

Provoking factors

Many patients have no obvious precipitating events before the development of the nephrotic syndrome, but non-specific upper respiratory tract infection is the commonest. More rarely, pollen, penicillin, milk allergy, poison oak, lymphoma and carcinoma may be culpable.

Susceptibility

There is a higher incidence of atopy among patients and their families than the normal population. One study has shown an increased incidence of HLA–B12.

Clinical course

Most patients present with the sudden onset of the nephrotic syndrome (see above). Mild hypertension is common and microscopic haematuria sometimes occurs. Renal function is slightly reduced in many patients and very rarely acute renal failure develops, usually after the injudicious use of diuretics. Infections, particularly pneumococcal peritonitis, used to be common during the nephrotic phase but are no longer a major threat to the patient.

Spontaneous remissions occurred in about 50 per cent of patients before the introduction of steroids. It was also recognised that patients who contracted measles while in hospital were effectively cured.

INVESTIGATIONS

The changes of the nephrotic syndrome, namely heavy proteinuria, low serum albumin and high cholesterol are found. The selectivity of urinary protein loss is a useful investigation in children. 'Selectivity' is a ratio of the clearance of a large molecule such as IgG to that of a small one such as transferrin. In children a ratio of the clearances of those two molecules of less than 0·1 is highly suggestive of minimal change nephropathy and it is unnecessary to proceed to renal biopsy. In adults the selectivity is rarely measured as there are many false positives and negatives. All adult patients require renal biopsy. The concentration of IgA and IgG tend to be low even during remission, and IgM levels are high.

TREATMENT

The treatment of oedema has already been described. Prednisolone induces a remission of the nephrotic syndrome in about 85–95 per cent of patients with MCN. Most go into remission in the first two weeks of therapy but it is worth continuing for eight weeks. Prednisolone should be started at 60 mg per day for four days and then reduced to 40 mg per day. This dose should be maintained until proteinuria ceases, when the prednisolone can be tailed off. Relapses occur in 70 per cent of patients usually within a few months of withdrawing prednisolone therapy. Relapses are very rare after three years. Each relapse should be treated as above. If frequent relapses occur or if remission can only be sustained by continuing an unacceptably high dose of prednisolone, cyclophosphamide 3 mg/kg/day for eight weeks may be used to prolong remission induced by steroids. Chlorambucil can also be used but azathioprine has no effect. The mean length of remission following a course of cyclophosphamide is 18 months.

Failure to respond to steroids may indicate an error in diagnosis. Early membranous nephropathy should not be confused providing the biopsy material is studied by immunofluorescent techniques (see below). Focal glomerulosclerosis may be almost impossible to diagnose on a small biopsy sample. A more common cause of failure to respond may be the continuing activity of whatever effect precipitated the disease. For example, patients in whom the disease is associated with carcinoma, lymphoma or tuberculosis will not respond until the underlying disease has been treated.

The long term prognosis of patients with MCN is excellent. Renal failure does not develop, but an occasional patient still dies of infection or the complications of treatment.

Focal glomerulosclerosis (FGS) (Focal and segmental glomerulosclerosis and hyalinosis)

PATHOLOGY

Light microscopy

In the early stages of the disease most glomeruli are normal. The earliest change is the development of sclerosis in some lobules of some juxtamedullary glomeruli. More and more glomeruli become affected with time. For this reason, the diagnosis may be difficult to make in the early stages, and a generous biopsy is essential. It is difficult to distinguish between FGS and old focal proliferative glomerulonephritis and sometimes the lesions induced by ischaemia are remarkably similar.

Electron microscopy

Epithelial cell foot process fusion is present. Abnormal glomeruli may show areas of sclerosis and collapse of the capillary loops. Electron dense material is often found in the mesangial matrix.

Immunofluorescent studies

IgM and C3 are deposited in areas of sclerosis.

CLINICAL FEATURES

Age

Onset may occur at any age but the most common is between 15 and 30.

Sex

It is slightly more common in males.

Provoking factors

The only known clinical association is with heroin addiction.

Frequency

The changes of FGS are found in 10–15 per cent of renal biopsies in most series of patients with nephrotic syndrome.

Clinical course

Most patients present with the nephrotic syndrome. The severity of proteinuria may fluctuate spontaneously. Renal failure with hypertension develop in the majority of patients, of whom 50 per cent are dead or on dialysis within eight to ten years. Severe proteinuria may persist even in the advanced stages of renal failure. As a result some patients become quite cachectic and dialysis may have to be instituted comparatively early. The pathological changes may recur in a transplanted kidney, and proteinuria may develop within hours of transplantation.

INVESTIGATIONS

The diagnosis is made by renal biopsy. There are no chemical tests that distinguish it from other causes of the nephrotic syndrome.

TREATMENT

Steroids and cyclophosphamide may temporarily reduce the severity of proteinuria in some patients, but it is doubtful if therapy has a long term beneficial effect.

Membranous nephropathy

PATHOLOGY

Light microscopy

The main abnormality is a thickening of the glomerular basement membrane (GBM) as shown in Figure 6.2a. There are regular projections of basement membrane material towards the epithelial side.

Electron microscopy

Projections of GBM which may be seen on light microscopy are confirmed on EM. Electron dense deposits lie between them on the epithelial side of the GBM. This is characteristic of membranous nephropathy.

Immunofluorescent studies

Regular deposits of immunoglobulin, usually IgG, and some complement components are found along the GBM (see Fig. 6.2b). Mesangial deposits are rarely seen.

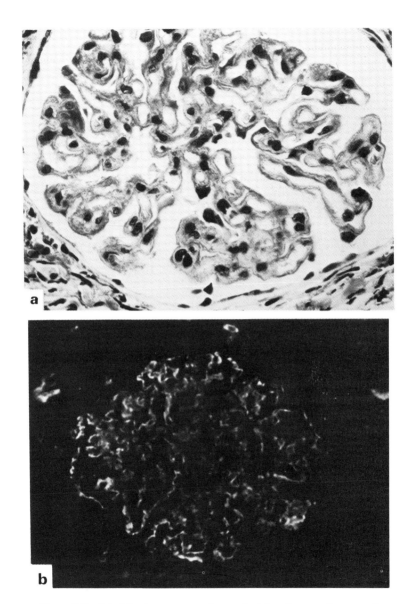

FIG. 6.2 (a) Membranous nephropathy showing no increase in number of cells, but the glomerular basement membrane is thickened. (b) Membranous nephropathy with regular fine deposits of C3 along glomerular basement membrane. IgG is deposited in a similar manner.

CLINICAL FEATURES

Age

Membranous nephropathy may present at any age but is most common between the ages of 35 and 45.

Sex

Males are affected more commonly.

Provoking factors

The cause is usually unknown, but these histological changes have been found in patients with tumours, particularly carcinoma, and with SLE. Some drugs may cause membranous nephropathy, the most common being gold and penicillamine. It is associated with HLA–DR3 in 70% of patients.

Frequency

It occurs in about 30–35 per cent of renal biopsies in adults.

Clinical course

Most patients present with either proteinuria or the nephrotic syndrome. Spontaneous remission occurs in 25 per cent, but about 40 per cent develop progressive renal failure with hypertension over five to ten years. The remainder have persistent urinary abnormalities with normal or reduced renal function. Patients presenting with the nephrotic syndrome have a worse prognosis than those who have proteinuria alone. Renal vein thrombosis, which may cause deterioration in renal function, flank pain and pulmonary emboli, appears to be particularly common in this form of glomerulopathy; at one time it was thought that renal vein thrombosis itself gave rise to the membranous nephropathy but this seems unlikely.

The lesion does not recur in transplanted kidneys but has developed in transplanted kidneys which had been grafted into patients in whom the cause of renal failure was not membranous nephropathy.

TREATMENT

A recent controlled trial of alternate day steroids for a three month period has suggested that this form of therapy may be of benefit in reducing proteinuria and preventing deterioration in renal function. Previous trials have shown no beneficial effect.

The proliferative glomerulopathies

ACUTE EXUDATIVE GLOMERULONEPHRITIS (POST-STREPTOCOCCAL GN)

Pathology

Light microscopy. Proliferation of endocapillary cells is the most prominent change. Neutrophils are present within capillary lumina. The basement membrane remains normal. In the more severe reactions, epithelial proliferation and crescent formation in a variable number of glomeruli may be seen.

Electron microscopy. Electron dense humps are found on the epithelial side of the basement membrane.

Immunofluorescent studies. Deposits of C3 are found but are often scanty. Immunoglobulins, most frequently IgG, are also present in the majority of patients. All deposits are along the basement membrane, but are not as regular as those seen in membranous nephropathy.

Clinical features

Age. The syndrome usually occurs in childhood, but can occur at any age.

Sex. Males are affected slightly more frequently than females.

Provoking factors. Classically, the disease develops ten days (range three to thirty days) after a streptococcal infection of the skin or throat. Only streptococci Lancefield group A of types 1, 2, 4, 12, 18, 25, 49, 55, 57 and 60 are associated with nephritis and are identified

more commonly in children. Other organisms such as staphylococci, pneumococci, Epstein–Barr virus and Coxsackie viral
infections are relatively more common in adults but sometimes no
cause can be found.

Incidence. This syndrome is much less common than it was, and the
reason for the decline is not known. It is relatively more common in
the developing countries, in which epidemics have been described.

Clinical cause. Patients present with the nephritic syndrome.
Sometimes proteinuria is severe enough to cause a fall in the serum
albumin concentration to give a mixed nephritic/nephrotic pattern
and this is thought to be associated with a worse prognosis,
particularly in adults. Treatment for acute renal failure is required
in a few patients. Most improve spontaneously. Haematuria and
proteinuria may persist for a few months or even some years. The
majority of children recover completely. The prognosis in adults is
slightly less favourable; patients with marked crescent formation
may develop irreversible renal failure in the short term and a
smaller proportion of adults who apparently recover from the acute
attack develop hypertension and renal failure some years later.
Thus long term follow-up is desirable.

Investigation

A raised ASO titre is found in about 85 per cent of patients.
Hypocomplementaemia (low C3) is present during the acute phase
and returns to normal after about six weeks.

Treatment

Penicillin should be given when the diagnosis is suspected to
eradicate residual streptococci but long term penicillin therapy is
unnecessary. Steroids may be helpful in patients with more florid
biopsy changes, but their effect remains unproven. Hypertension,
fluid overload and renal failure should be treated as described in
Chapter 10.

MESANGIOCAPILLARY GLOMERULONEPHRITIS (MCGN) (MEMBRANOPROLIFERATIVE GN, LOBULAR GN, HYPOCOMPLEMENTAEMIC GN)

Pathology

Light microscopy. Thickening of the GBM, associated with mesangial cell proliferation, is the hallmark of this type of glomerulopathy. The GBM appears to be split by an intrusion of the mesangial matrix.

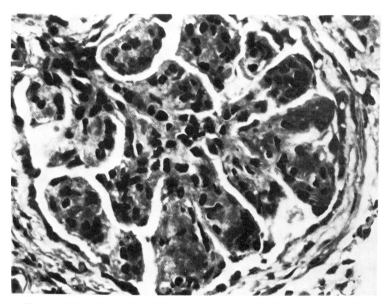

FIG. 6.3 Mesangiocapillary glomerulonephritis showing the glomerular tufts arranged in a lobular manner and that many capillary loops are obliterated.

Electron microscopy. This confirms the extension of mesangial matrix into the GBM. There are two main types distinguished by the site of electron dense deposits. In type 1 these are subendothelial and in type 2 (dense deposit disease) large bands of electron dense deposits are found within the GBM.

Immunofluorescent studies. The most prominent and consistent finding is coarse granular deposition of C3 round the peripheral capillaries of each lobule of the glomerular tuft. IgG and IgM are sometimes present in a similar distribution.

Clinical features

Age. MCGN usually presents in patients between the ages of 5 and 30.

Sex. Both sexes are equally affected.

Provoking factors and associations. The onset often follows an upper respiratory tract infection from which the organism is rarely identified. Patients with partial lipodystrophy and circulating C3 nephritic factor (see below) are particularly prone to develop this form of glomerulopathy as do some patients with an infected atrioventricular shunt (usually due to *Staphylococcus albus*) or infective endocarditis.

Clinical course. The most common presentation is with the nephrotic syndrome. However, almost any of the presentations described earlier in this chapter may occur. A minority present with a nephritic syndrome and transient renal failure from which recovery is never complete. Progressive renal failure is the rule, but a minority of patients have persistent proteinuria with normal renal function for several years. Hypertension is common and may be difficult to control. Anaemia is sometimes more marked than expected for the degree of renal failure. Prognosis is slightly worse than that of FGS and membranous nephropathy, 50 per cent being dead or on dialysis within six to eight years. The same histological changes may occur in transplanted kidneys and recurrences are particularly common in patients with the dense deposit variety of MCGN (type 2).

Investigation

Eighty per cent of patients with these biopsy changes have a reduced blood concentration of C3. C4 levels are usually normal. A circulating factor, C3 nephritic factor, is capable of splitting C3 to C3b and C3a *in vitro*. Neither the concentration of C3 nor that of C3 nephritic factor correlate with disease activity. In fact, these abnormalities may pre-date the onset of renal disease by several years because they are also found in patients with partial lipodystrophy whether or not they have renal disease. It is probable that a low C3 level predisposes to this type of nephritis.

Treatment

There is no specific effective treatment other than the detection and management of any precipitating cause in those patients in whom it can be identified. The complications will require treatment as they arise.

RAPIDLY PROGRESSIVE GLOMERULONEPHRITIS (RPGN) (CRESCENTIC NEPHRITIS)

Pathology

Light microscopy. The dominant abnormality of this form of nephritis is the presence of cellular proliferation outside the glomerular tuft but within Bowman's capsule to form the characteristic crescent (Fig. 6.4a). The proliferating cells may be either epithelial cells or macrophages or both. RPGN is defined as the presence of crescents in over 70 per cent of glomeruli. Endocapillary proliferation may also be present in some patients. Interstitial and tubular changes are always found.

Electron microscopy. Patients with associated endocapillary proliferation may have some endothelial, mesangial or subepithelial electron dense deposits. Destruction of capillary loops by proliferation of epithelial cells may be apparent. Fibrin deposits may be seen.

Immunofluorescent studies. The crescents stain for fibrin, unless present for more than a few weeks. The other immunofluorescent findings depend on the aetiology. Linear deposits of immuno-globulin or complement may be found in patients with anti-GBM disease, including Goodpasture's syndrome (Fig. 6.4b); granular deposits are found in subacute infective endocarditis (SIE) and systemic lupus erythematosus (SLE). Deposits may be absent in patients with polyarteritis nodosa or Wegener's granulomatosis

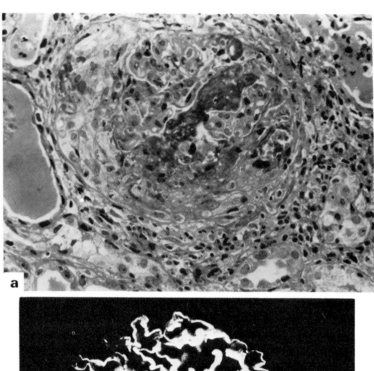

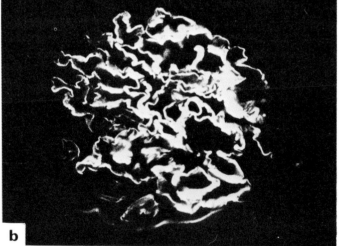

FIG. 6.4 (a) Crescentic nephritis showing the remnants of the glomerular tuft surrounded by a 'crescent' which consists of proliferating epithelial cells and macrophages and contains fibrin.
(b) Antiglomerular basement membrane disease. Some patients with crescentic nephritis have linear deposits of IgG along the basement membrane. Most of these patients have Goodpastures syndrome, i.e. associated haemoptysis.

although this is not an invariable rule; granular deposits of immunoglobulin, particularly IgA, may be present in patients with Henoch–Schonlein purpura. Thus the immunofluorescent findings may be of diagnostic help in patients with multi-system disease (Table 6.2).

TABLE 6.2 Glomerular immunofluorescent changes and systemic diseases.

Disease	Pattern	Principal immunoglobulin	C3	Fibrin*
SLE	Granular mesangial and or capillary loop	IgG	+	+
SIE	Granular mesangial	IgG	+	+
PAN	—	—	—	+
Wegener's	—	—	—	+
HSP	Granular mesangial	IgA	+	+
Goodpasture's syndrome	Linear capillary loop	IgG	+	+

*Usually in recently formed crescents.

Clinical features

Age. Patients usually present between the ages of 30 and 60.

Sex. Two males are affected for every female.

Associated diseases. This syndrome often appears as part of one of several systemic diseases, of which polyarteritis nodosa is the most common. It also occurs in Wegener's granulomatosis, SLE, SIE, Goodpasture's syndrome, post-streptococcal glomerulonephritis or Henoch–Schonlein purpura. However, renal involvement may be the only indication of disease.

Clinical course. The onset is usually insidious with the patients complaining of increasing tiredness and oedema. There may be some symptoms referrable to another organ such as haemoptysis which may occur in both Goodpasture's syndrome and polyarteritis nodosa. On examination, the patient is anaemic, blood pressure is either normal or slightly elevated and oedema is present. Proteinuria and haematuria are invariably found and red cell and granular casts usually detected on microscopy. Oliguria or anuria are often present by the time the diagnosis is made. An acute nephritic onset suggests endocapillary proliferation such as is associated with streptococcal infection. Most patients are either dead or on dialysis within six months. The fewer the number of crescents present on a renal biopsy the better the prognosis, whatever the pathogenetic mechanism.

Investigations

Those relating to the detection of systemic disease will be described in Chapter 7. There are no specific immunological or biochemical abnormalities in this type of glomerulopathy.

Treatment

If the patient is anuric by the time the diagnosis is made and is suitable for regular dialysis, then this should be started. If the urine volume is greater than 400 ml/24 hours, treatment may be of value. Steroids given as pulses of methylprednisolone 1 g intravenously on alternate days, together with oral prednisolone 40 mg/day plus cyclophosphamide 3 mg/kg/day and heparin or ancrod (which effectively defibrinates the patient) have been used. More recently regular plasma exchange has given some promising results both in Goodpasture's disease and in acute immune complex induced crescentic nephritis. The efficacy of these forms of therapy has not as yet been substantiated by controlled trials.

FOCAL PROLIFERATIVE GLOMERULONEPHRITIS

Pathology

Light microscopy. Focal proliferation means that some glomeruli show cellular, usually mesangial, proliferation. Other glomeruli are completely normal. The proliferation within a glomerulus is often segmental, i.e. confined to one or more of the lobules which make up the glomerular tuft. Epithelial proliferation is sometimes present (Fig. 6.5a).

Electron microscopy. This confirms the cellular proliferation seen on light microscopy. The detailed findings depend on the underlying disease process; see below.

Immunofluorescent studies. Linear staining of IgG is found in the occasional patient with anti-GBM disease, granular deposits of IgG and C3 in patients with immune complex disease and no deposits in the majority of patients presenting with polyarteritis nodosa. Berger's disease (see below) is associated with mesangial deposits of IgA and C3; IgG is sometimes seen as well (Fig. 6.5b).

Clinical features

Age. Patients usually present between the ages of 15 and 40.

Sex. Males are more commonly affected than females.

Associated diseases. These are the same as for RPGN; there is a continuum between the two histological types. The more severe renal involvement is associated with a greater number of crescents.

Clinical course. The most common presentation in patients who do not have a systemic disease such as SLE or polyarteritis nodosa (PAN) is recurrent frank haematuria. It almost always affects young men who have marked macroscopic but painless haematuria 24 to 48 hours after an upper respiratory tract infection or less commonly following exercise. This may happen repeatedly. It is important to recognise this syndrome and confirm the diagnosis by renal biopsy since a firm diagnosis may remove the need for further IVU's, cystoscopies, retrograde pyelograms and arteriograms. The association of these symptoms with mesangial IgA deposits was first described by Berger and the prognosis is usually good with no deterioration in renal function over several years. A small proportion of patients develop significant proteinuria, hypertension and renal failure. These patients may have a recurrence of the disease in a transplanted kidney.

Apart from this well-defined group, most patients with focal proliferative glomerulonephritis present with proteinuria. The

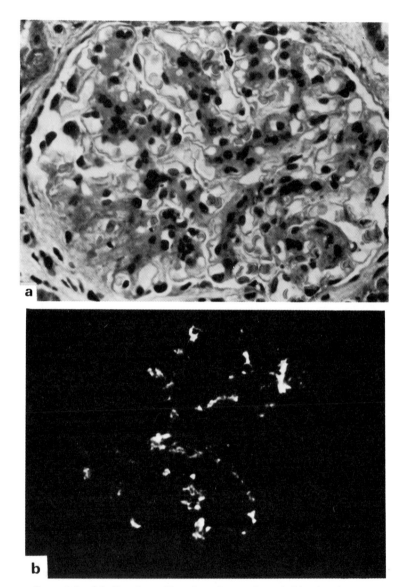

FIG. 6.5 (a) Focal proliferative glomerulonephritis showing too many mesangial cells in parts of this glomerulus. Other glomeruli in the biopsy are entirely normal.

(b) Mesangial IgA disease. Many patients, but not all, with focal proliferative glomerulonephritis have deposits of IgA in the mesangium.

nephrotic syndrome and hypertension are rare and progression to renal failure is unusual.

Treatment

Since the renal prognosis is good, no specific renal treatment is required. If a systemic disease is present, this may require treatment as outlined in Chapter 7.

MESANGIAL PROLIFERATIVE GLOMERULONEPHRITIS

This is an even more heterogenous group with no clear clinical picture. Some patients have resolving post-streptococcal glomerulonephritis, others present with the nephrotic syndrome and have only minor degrees of mesangial proliferation with negative immunofluorescent studies; these patients respond to prednisolone in the same way as patients with minimal change nephropathy. The overall prognosis of patients with mesangial proliferation is excellent.

PATHOGENETIC MECHANISMS OF GLOMERULOPATHY

The pathological classification of glomerulopathy does not distinguish diseases. Each histological group appears to be made up of patients who have a variety of clinical presentations, associated diseases and prognoses. The advances in our understanding of the way in which these histological changes develop have largely resulted from the study of animal models of glomerulonephritis and immunofluorescent studies of renal biopsies. However, our knowledge is not yet complete enough to offer an alternative pathogenetic classification.

Two pathogenetic mechanisms are now well established.

Anti-glomerular basement membrane antibody

Animal model

'Nephrotoxic nephritis' is easily produced; glomerular preparations of rabbits' kidneys can be made and injected into another animal such as a sheep which produces an antibody in high titre to the rabbit glomerular basement membrane. This antibody when injected into a rabbit will cause a two stage glomerulonephritis.

Stage 1: Heterologous phase. The sheep antibody fixes to the rabbit's GBM and within two to three days proteinuria develops. The sheep antibody can be detected on the rabbit GBM by immunofluorescent techniques. The histological changes which appear at this time are of mild endocapillary proliferation. Their action is dependent on complement. The amount of antibody fixed to the glomerular basement membrane may be as little as 15µg/g of kidney tissue.

Stage 2: Autologous phase. The rabbit develops an antibody to the sheep IgG and this also fixes on the glomerular basement membrane at about the sixth day. By the tenth day a fulminating crescentic nephritis is produced and the rabbit dies of renal failure in two weeks. This reaction has been shown to be markedly reduced if the animal is depleted of polymorph neutrophils or if the circulating fibrinogen is removed by the administration of ancrod. Therefore, both polymorphs and the coagulation system are important mediators of injury in the autologous phase of nephrotoxic nephritis. Rather surprisingly, decomplementing the animal with cobra venom does not ameliorate the disease.

The antibody—whether heterologous sheep anti-GBM or autologous rabbit anti-sheep IgG—can be detected by immunofluorescent techniques as a fine linear band along the GBM. This is relevant to the study of human renal biopsies.

Human anti-GBM nephritis

Linear IgG on the GBM can be demonstrated in between three and five per cent of human renal biopsies. The pathogenicity of this antibody has been confirmed by eluting it from the kidney following nephrectomy and injecting it into a squirrel monkey which then develops a similar nephritis. Furthermore, the titre of anti-GBM antibody in the patient's serum rises after bilateral nephrectomy, which is indirect evidence of the specificity of the antibody to the GBM. Lastly, in about 15 per cent of patients with this type of nephritis who undergo transplantation, recurrent disease develops in the transplanted kidney.

CLINICAL FEATURES

Age

The peak incidence is between 15 and 50 years.

Sex

Males are affected four times more commonly than females.

Provoking factors

About 60 per cent of patients have a preceding history of an upper respiratory tract infection. Unusually heavy exposure to hydrocarbons is also much more common in this group of patients. HLA DR2 is present in about 90 per cent of patients which is significantly more than the general population.

Clinical course

Goodpasture's syndrome. This is the association of renal failure due to crescentic nephritis with haemoptysis which may predate evidence of renal involvement by months or even years. The haemoptysis may be trivial and only found by looking for haemosiderin-laden macrophages in the sputum or may be so severe as to threaten the patient's life.

Renal presentation ranges from mild proteinuria with normal renal function to oliguric renal failure. The urine contains protein, red cells and red cell casts. Oedema is often present but the blood pressure is either normal or only moderately raised. Unfortunately renal failure is usually advanced by the time of diagnosis. Anaemia may be profound and the red cells are both hypochromic and microcytic. The serum iron is usually reduced.

Anti-GBM disease without pulmonary involvement. About 25 per cent of patients with linear IgG on their biopsies have no evidence of pulmonary involvement. The majority present with renal failure due to crescentic nephritis. A minority have only mild renal failure and proteinuria which is sometimes severe enough to cause oedema. This presentation is relatively more common in women.

PATHOLOGY

Light microscopy

The changes of focal proliferation and crescentic nephritis are usually found. Many patients have more than 70 per cent crescents.

Immunofluorescent studies

All biopsies share the finding of linear deposition of IgG on the GBM. About 75 per cent of patients also have linear deposits of C3.

Hypothesis of pathogenesis of Goodpasture's syndrome

Lung damage is caused by virus infection or hydrocarbon exposure revealing new antigens to which patients of a particular HLA-D group make antibodies. The antibody cross reacts with the GBM causing nephritis similar to that seen in animals with nephrotoxic nephritis.

TREATMENT

If the patient is already anuric, no treatment is likely to restore useful renal function. Therefore, early diagnosis is essential. In the patients who are not oliguric, prednisolone and cytotoxic agents combined with anticoagulants and repeated plasma exchange (which removes circulating antibodies against the GBM as well as mediators of tissue damage) appear to arrest further renal damage and permit partial recovery of renal function. In many patients the disease itself is self-limiting and treatment can be tailed off after a few months. If the patient is already anuric it is best to start regular dialysis treatment and to consider transplantation after the anti-GBM levels have fallen to normal. Lung haemorrhage is readily controlled by plasma exchange.

Immune complex nephritis

This is the second well established mechanism known to cause renal damage.

ANIMAL MODEL

Acute serum sickness

The injection of any heterologous protein into an animal causes the production of antibodies directed against it. The treatment of patients thought liable to develop tetanus or diphtheria with antitoxin raised in another animal was often followed by a period of sickness which started seven to ten days after the injection and consisted of fever, proteinuria, joint pains and myocarditis. Animal models have shown that the symptoms occur when antibody is produced and residual circulating antigen is bound to it. The symptoms resolve a few days after all traces of antigen—whether combined with antibody or free—have disappeared from circulation. Once this has happened, free antibody can be detected. The pathological changes in the kidney of these animals is strikingly similar to acute exudative glomerulonephritis, i.e. endocapillary proliferation, neutrophil infiltration and in the more severely ill, focal necrosis and crescent formation. On electron microscopy, epithelial humps can be identified.

The possibility that immune complexes (antigen–antibody combinations) might be the cause of these changes was substantiated by the presence of antigen in the glomerulus, albeit in very small amounts, together with and in the same distribution as immunoglobulin and C3.

Chronic serum sickness

Rabbits given a fixed dose of bovine serum albumin (BSA) daily for several weeks may have one of four responses.

1. No antibody to BSA is produced; these animals remain well.

2. A brisk antibody response ensues; these animals also remain well unless the production of antibody decreases.

3. Intermediate antibody response occurs but free antigen can still be detected; these animals develop glomerulopathies which resemble membranous nephropathy or diffuse proliferative glomerulonephritis sometimes with crescents. The circulating complexes are small and deposits are found on the epithelial side of the GBM.

4. Slightly greater antibody response occurs and no free antigen

is detectable; these animals also have evidence of glomerulopathy but the changes are those of a focal proliferative glomerulonephritis. The circulating immune complexes are larger and the deposits are found in the mesangium and on the subendothelial side of the GBM.

Thus, one experimental protocol may induce focal or mesangial proliferation, membranous nephropathy, or diffuse proliferative glomerulonephritis with or without crescents. It should be emphasised that the majority of animals do not develop any glomerular abnormality. The liability of a particular animal to form complexes which cause renal damage seems to depend on the adequacy of its immune response. Work in mice has confirmed that strains which produce antibody of low avidity or have an inefficient reticulo-endothelial function are more likely to suffer spontaneous immune complex disease, in which the antigen is frequently of viral origin.

CLINICAL HALLMARKS OF IMMUNE COMPLEX DISEASE

Tests of circulating immune complexes

Numerous and ingenious tests have been designed to demonstrate circulating immune complexes. Unfortunately, no single test has proved reliable and none is established in routine clinical use.

Activation of complement cascade

Activation of the classical pathway of the complement cascade occurs as a result of immune complex activation of the first component of complement (Clq). Therefore, the demonstration of reduced concentrations of C4 and C3 in the blood is good indirect evidence of circulating immune complexes. Such changes are found in the blood of patients with nephritis associated with the active phase of SLE, subacute infective endocarditis, essential cryoglobulinaemia and acute exudative glomerulopathy. It should be noted that the low C3 concentration found in patients with MCGN is usually associated with normal C4 and is a result of activation of the alternate complement pathway by C3 nephritic factor.

Mixed cryoglobulinaemia

The finding of circulating mixed cryoglobulins is good evidence of immune complex disease provided that monoclonal immuno-globulin overproduction has been excluded.

Renal biopsy

The demonstration of an immunoglobulin and/or C3 distributed in all glomeruli in a granular or lumpy pattern in the mesangium or along the GBM is thought to be pathognomonic of immune complex disease.

Absolute proof that a particular glomerulopathy is caused by immune complex deposition can only be obtained if the antigen can be demonstrated in the same distribution as the immunoglobulin or if the immunoglobulin eluted from the kidney or biopsy material is specific for a certain antigen. Since the antigen can rarely be identified this is seldom possible.

IMPLICATIONS FOR TREATMENT

Unfortunately, although immune complex nephropathy is common and its pathogenicity established, these discoveries have not revolutionised the treatment of patients largely because the antigen cannot be identified. Where this is possible (see below), elimination of the source of antigen may lead to remarkable recovery in renal function. Anti-inflammatory agents such as prednisolone have been tried, usually unsuccessfully, in many forms of chronic glomerulopathies.

AETIOLOGY OF GLOMERULOPATHIES

Infections

Many infections, including viral, bacterial and protozoal, have been shown to cause immune complex nephritis. Perhaps malarial nephropathy is the most common in the world (see pages 140–42).

Tumours

Almost any tumour may cause the formation of immune complexes. It is more common in malignant tumours.

Drugs

Penicillamine, gold, troxidone and mercury have all been shown to cause glomerulonephropathies.

Autoantibodies

DNA, thyroglobulin and renal brush border antigens have been implicated.

CONCLUSIONS

The glomerulopathies have been the subject of intense epidemiological and experimental study over the last two decades. Only minimal change nephropathy can be effectively treated, but the therapy used is not without its own danger. Studies of renal biopsies have also enabled clinicians to divide groups of patients into those with a good, bad or very bad prognosis but the course of an individual patient may differ strikingly from the group to which the patient has been assigned. The study of the pathogenetic mechanisms has given most help in the management of patients with the rare form of nephritis associated with anti-GBM disease. The managament of patients with immune complex disease has not been advanced, primarily because the search for the precipitating antigen has been unsuccessful in all but a handful of patients. At present, the old advice that one should avoid harming patients by any treatment offered, remains the most applicable.

POINTS OF EMPHASIS

- The nephrotic syndrome comprises proteinuria of such magnitude as to cause hypoproteinaemia resulting in oedema formation.

- The nephrotic syndrome is associated with an increased liability to infection and accelerated atheroma formation.

- Irrespective of the diagnosis, when renal function permits, adults with a nephrotic syndrome should take 1·5 g/kg bodyweight of protein daily but children require much more.

- Diuretic therapy in the nephrotic syndrome requires careful monitoring because an excessive reduction in the circulating blood volume may aggravate renal failure.

- The management of the nephritic syndrome includes fluid restriction because of the increase in the total circulating fluid volume.

- Renal biopsy is usually indicated in the nephrotic syndrome to establish a pathological diagnosis.

- The pathological classification of glomerulopathies does not distinguish disease. Each histological group comprises patients with a variety of associated diseases and prognoses.

- Minimal change nephropathy (MCN) is the cause of the nephrotic syndrome in 90 per cent of children and 25 per cent of adults.

- About 90 per cent of patients with MCN respond to steroid therapy but many will relapse when steroids are withdrawn.

- 25 per cent of patients with membranous nephropathy undergo spontaneous remission; the prognosis is poorer in those presenting with a nephrotic syndrome.

- Most children presenting with an acute post-streptococcal nephritic syndrome recover completely.

- The prognosis is less favourable in adults, a few of whom have a proliferative glomerulonephritis of such severity as to cause irreversible renal failure. Others may develop hypertension and renal failure several years later and long term follow-up is desirable.

● In most patients, the cause of mesangiocapillary glomerulonephritis is obscure. Progression to renal failure is the rule and management is symptomatic.

● Rapidly progressive glomerulonephritis is often part of a systemic disorder such as PAN. Most patients progress to end stage renal failure within six months. Combined anticoagulation, immunosuppression and plasma exchange may be effective in the management of Goodpasture's syndrome and in acute immune complex induced crescentic nephritis.

● Focal proliferative glomerulonephritis may be associated with the same systemic disorders as rapidly progressive glomerulonephritis.

CHAPTER 7

The kidney and systemic disease

INTRODUCTION

The kidney is involved in a great variety of systemic disorders. In some the renal abnormality may threaten the life of the patient; in others it may help in the diagnosis of an otherwise obscure disorder because there are accurate descriptions of the renal abnormalities associated with many systemic diseases. The following is an account of some such diseases.

THE KIDNEY AND COLLAGEN DISORDERS

Systemic lupus erythematosus (SLE)

Clinical features

Age. The onset usually occurs between 15 and 45.

Sex. SLE is eight times more common in women.

Less than ten per cent of patients present with renal manifestations of SLE. Rashes, joint pains or serositis are more common presenting complaints. However, renal involvement is the most important factor in the evolution of the disease in over half the patients, and is often apparent within one year of diagnosis. The two most common renal presentations are proteinuria, which may be discovered on routine urinalysis, and the nephrotic syndrome. Acute renal failure is rare. Hypertension and chronic renal failure develop in about 50 per cent of patients, but are rarely present when renal involvement is diagnosed. The urine usually contains red cells and red cell granular casts as well as protein. Renal function varies widely on presentation but the creatinine clearance is usually near normal early in the disease. Unfortunately, the clinical findings and tests of renal function are of little help in determining the outcome although the development of hypertension, nephrotic syndrome and renal failure are indications of poor prognosis. Most studies have shown that the renal prognosis depends upon the changes found on renal biopsy. The management of renal involvement depends upon the nature of the pathological process. It follows that a renal biopsy should be performed in all patients with proteinuria of more than 0·5 g/day, an abnormal urinalysis (red cells or red cell casts) or reduced renal function unless there is a specific contraindication (see page 38).

Pathology

The changes seen on renal biopsy can be divided into four groups.

No significant change

Most glomeruli look normal on light microscopy or show minor mesangial cell proliferation. No diffuse deposits of immunoglobulin or complement are found on immunofluorescent studies.

Clinical correlation. These patients have either no or minimal proteinuria. The creatinine clearance and blood pressure are usually normal and their renal prognosis is excellent.

Focal proliferative and mesangial proliferative glomerulitis

Light microscopy. Glomeruli may be normal or contain areas of endocapillary proliferation. Other glomeruli may have prominent mesangial matrix and proliferation of mesangial cells. Epithelial proliferation is rare. Tubular and interstitial changes are minimal.

Electron microscopy. Dense deposits are found in the mesangial areas and not around the capillary loops.

Immunofluorescent studies. Mesangial deposits of immunoglobulin

(IgG usually with IgA and IgM) and complement components are found in all glomeruli.

Clinical correlation. Proteinuria is the main finding, but it is rarely serious enough to cause nephrotic syndrome. Hypertension is also rare. The renal prognosis is usually good. These changes are found in about 30 per cent of patients with renal lupus.

Membranous nephropathy

The pathological change on light and electron microscopy and the immunofluorescent findings are exactly the same as those described for idiopathic membranous nephropathy (see Chapter 6). Some patients may also have a few mesangial deposits and areas of focal proliferation.

Clinical correlation. Patients present with proteinuria or the nephrotic syndrome. The renal prognosis is also the same as that of idiopathic membranous nephropathy. Membranous changes are found in about ten per cent of biopsies of patients with lupus nephritis.

Diffuse lupus glomerulonephritis

Light microscopy. All glomeruli show a proliferative reaction. Areas of focal and/or fibrinoid necrosis may be found. Some epithelial proliferation is common, but widespread crescent formation is rare. The pathognomonic lesion of lupus nephritis, i.e. a haematoxyphil body, is also rarely seen. Areas of interstitial and tubular damage are common, and reflect the gravity of this type of nephritis (Fig. 7.1).

Electron microscopy. Dense deposits are found in the mesangium, and around the capillary loops, where they may occur on both the endothelial and epithelial side of the basement membrane.

Immunofluorescent studies. Deposits of immunoglobulins (mostly IgG) and complement components are found in the same distribution as the dense deposits seen on electron microscopy.

Clinical correlation. Although more females are affected than

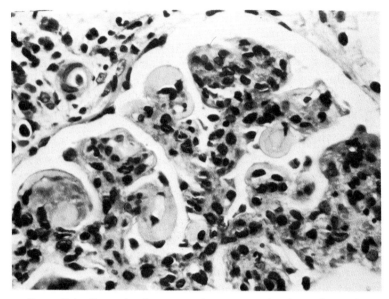

FIG. 7.1 Systemic lupus erythematosus showing glomerulus containing an excess number of mesangial cells, double contours of many capillary loops and a hyaline thrombus.

males, this type of lupus nephritis is relatively more common in men than are the other histological categories. Nephrotic syndrome, hypertension and renal failure are all more common, and progression to terminal renal failure is frequent. Occasionally, diffuse changes are found in patients whose only renal abnormality is minimal proteinuria.

INVESTIGATION AND DIAGNOSIS

The diagnosis of SLE has traditionally been made by fulfilling the clinical and laboratory criteria defined by the American Rheumatology Association. An easier diagnostic criterion is the finding of a raised *DNA binding* titre using double stranded DNA as antigen. This is raised during periods of clinical activity in all patients with lupus nephritis as well as many who have clinically inactive disease. It is not, therefore, a good guide for treatment. Drug induced lupus is not associated with a raised DNA binding, and renal involvement is extremely rare.

All patients have a *positive ANF*, but this may occur in many patients who have no other evidence of SLE. Therefore, the association of a positive ANF with proteinuria does not in itself establish the diagnosis of lupus nephritis. *C3 and C4 concentrations* are usually reduced during the active phase of the disease indicating activation of the classical complement pathway. *Mixed cryoglobulinaemia* is also common during active phases of the disease and represents circulating immune complexes, which can be readily detected by *immune complex assays*.

Unfortunately, there is no simple laboratory test which regularly reflects the degree of disease activity. Changes in renal function as measured by creatinine clearance or serum creatinine remain the best guide to the efficacy of treatment; regular re-biopsy of the patient's kidney may also give a good guide as to what proportion of the renal lesion is potentially reversible. Re-biopsy may also be useful to ensure that the patient has not changed from one histological group to another. Fortunately, this happens comparatively rarely.

TREATMENT

Focal and membranous nephritis

These have good renal prognoses and usually no specific therapy is required. Treatment is aimed at controlling the symptoms caused by involvement of other organs. Rarely, a patient with these renal lesions may suffer a progressive decline of renal function, and if so re-biopsy is indicated in case there has been a deterioration in histological category to diffuse lupus nephritis.

Diffuse lupus nephritis

Steroid therapy. There have been no properly controlled clinical trials of steroid therapy in the treatment of lupus nephritis. However, comparison with earlier series and clinical experience have convinced most nephrologists that high dose prednisolone (over 40 mg/day) improves the renal prognosis. More recently, intravenous pulses of methyl prednisolone in doses up to 1 g given on alternate days have also been used over shorter periods with good results. The dose of prednisolone should be titrated against changes in renal function using the minimum dose which maintains

renal function. Relapses should be treated by increasing to 40 mg/
day or by giving pulses of methyl prednisolone 1 g on alternate
days up to a total of 5 g.

Cytotoxic agents. Cyclophosphamide and azathioprine have almost
always been used together with prednisolone but the results of trials
are contradictory. It is probable that azathioprine 2 mg/kg/day does
enable the use of a lower dose of steroids to achieve the same
clinical response, and this has become the practice of many
nephrologists. Cyclophosphamide has a similar role, but its
unwanted effects are less acceptable, particularly hair loss in women
and the longer term bladder complications.

Plasma exchange has been reported to reduce clinical activity in
patients with evidence of circulating immune complexes. It is
expensive to perform and its place in the treatment of lupus
nephritis remains unknown.

Anticoagulants are not used except in the rare patients with
crescentic nephritis.

Chloroquine has no established place in the treatment of lupus
nephritis.

PROGNOSIS

Patients with SLE appear to have a much better prognosis now than
in the 1950's. The reason for this is obscure; it may be due to
diagnosing patients with milder forms of disease, better treatment
or a change in the severity of the disease. Fifty per cent of patients
with *diffuse* lupus glomerulonephritis survived for 18 months in the
1950's, for three years in the 1960's when high dose prednisolone
was used and for ten years in the 1970's. The renal prognosis for
membranous and focal lupus nephritis is better, the patients usually
dying of a non-renal cause. Complications of treatment are
common. Opportunistic infections by viruses, bacteria and fungi
occur and are the cause of some deaths. Avascular necrosis of the
head of the femur may develop and require surgical replacement of
the joint. Spontaneous remissions and exacerbations are frequent,
often for no apparent reason except in those patients with the
classical association with exposure to sunlight. Therefore,

treatment should be reviewed regularly and kept at the minimum required to control symptoms and maintain renal function.

Polyarteritis nodosa (PAN)

PAN is a disease of unknown aetiology in which medium-sized arteries or arterioles are involved in an inflammatory reaction. Any vessel may be affected so that the clinical consequences are variable.

PATHOGENESIS

The aetiology of this disease is unknown. In some series from Europe and the Eastern part of the USA, a number of patients were found to have hepatitis B antigenaemia. This has not been confirmed in the UK.

CLINICAL FINDINGS

The disease mostly affects middle aged men although it may occur in patients of any age and either sex. The classical presentation comprises fever, malaise and symptoms attributable to involvement of several organs. Common features include purpuric rashes, joint pains, lung involvement and mononeuritis multiplex. A similar syndrome may be provoked by drugs (see Chapter 13).

RENAL PRESENTATION

PAN may cause almost any renal presentation. The most common is acute renal failure with proteinuria and haematuria. Proteinuria is rarely sufficiently large to cause nephrotic syndrome. Hypertension is quite common. Much more rarely, the patient may present with an obstructive uropathy due to an arteritis causing narrowing of the ureteric lumen.

PATHOLOGY

Light microscopy

The glomeruli may show a great variety of changes ranging between focal proliferation, focal necrosis of some tufts and widespread crescent formation. Tubular and interstitial changes may be severe. Sometimes, an artery or arteriole may be included in the biopsy which shows the changes characteristic of PAN. These are of an inflammatory exudate involving neutrophils and mononuclear cells affecting all the layers of the artery, although the process probably starts in the adventitia. However, only a minority of arteries are involved and the diagnosis is rarely made in this way.

Immunofluorescent studies

The immunofluorescent findings are variable. Usually no diffuse deposits of immunoglobin or complement are found in the glomeruli. Fibrin is often present in crescents and some of the glomerular tufts. In a minority of patients diffuse deposits of immunoglobilin and complement are found; these patients often have circulating cryoglobulins.

INVESTIGATION AND DIAGNOSIS

The firm diagnosis depends on demonstrating the pathological changes of an affected vessel. Blind biopsies of the pectoral muscle or the testes have been recommended but are rarely rewarding. Arteriography offers a better chance, because many more vessels can be examined and aneurysms, typical of polyarteritis affecting medium-sized arteries, can sometimes be identified. Neutrophilia is usually present, but eosinophilia is less common though of more significance. Complement levels are normal. The diagnosis often rests on clinical suspicion. The combination of a disease affecting the kidney and another organ, the biopsy findings of focal proliferation or crescentic nephritis without diffuse deposits of immunoglobulin or complement is highly suggestive and is sufficient to undertake a trial of treatment.

TREATMENT

Steroids are the mainstay of treatment and frequently lead to an improvement in renal function and an abatement of symptoms such as rash, cough, breathlessness or joint pain. High doses of prednisolone may be required. Azathioprine and cyclophosphamide appear to be effective in individual patients. Plasma exchange and/or anticoagulant therapy may help in patients with crescentic nephritis. No satisfactory controlled trials have been conducted to substantiate any treatment of the renal lesions of PAN.

PROGNOSIS

The absence of a serological marker means that the diagnosis is made at post mortem in about 25 per cent of patients. Untreated patients normally die within one year, but treatment appears to increase survival so that 50 per cent of patients now survive five years. Disease activity may abate spontaneously, and recurrences occur, sometimes after several years.

Wegener's granulomatosis

This is a disease of granulomatous and necrotising lesions of the respiratory tract. The majority of patients also have glomerulonephritis which is indistinguishable from that of polyarteritis nodosa.

Rheumatoid arthritis (RA)

RA primarily affects joints. Other organs may be involved, but the kidneys are rarely affected directly. Renal involvement occurs as a complication which may be due to amyloid (see below) or drug therapy. Analgesics are an essential part of treatment and therefore analgesic nephropathy is more common than in the general population. Gold and penicillamine are also used in the treatment, and may cause proteinuria and the nephrotic syndrome for which a renal biopsy should be performed. If amyloid is found, the drugs can be continued but if the changes of membranous nephropathy are seen, treatment with the offending drug should be stopped. Drug-induced proteinuria usually disappears within a few months.

Systemic sclerosis

Serious renal involvement in systemic sclerosis is rare. Mild proteinuria occurs quite often but is of little significance. Very occasionally acute renal failure develops. This is due to proliferation of the media and intima of renal arterioles indistinguishable from the changes seen in malignant hypertension. Indeed, hypertension does develop in these patients, but this is the consequence and not the cause of the arteriolar changes. Any recovery of renal function is exceptional but has been reported. Vasodilator drugs such as diazoxide may help. Dialysis has been attempted but the gross thickening of the skin makes vascular access difficult and the use of the subcutaneous fistula impossible.

THE KIDNEY AND INFECTION

The kidney as a site of infection has been discussed in Chapter 4. It may also be affected in various ways by infection in other parts of the body.

Acute tubular necrosis

This is described in more detail in Chapter 8. Septicaemia and other acute infections are the cause of ATN in about ten per cent of patients with this disorder and a contributing factor in many more. Recovery of renal function almost invariably follows elimination of infection, if this can be achieved.

Acute interstitial nephritis

See Chapter 4. Distant infection may also cause renal failure due to acute interstitial nephritis. This may be more common than is realised because renal biopsies are seldom performed in these circumstances and the natural history is very similar to acute tubular necrosis. Post mortems performed early in the century established the association with scarlet fever and other acute infections. More recently it has been described in association with Legionnaires' disease.

Amyloid

Chronic infection, particularly apparently inactive pulmonary tuberculosis, was until recently the commonest cause of amyloid seen in Britain. Rheumatoid arthritis is now the most common cause. Secondary amyloid, with the exception of that due to myeloma (Table 7.1), is made of polymerised amyloid A fibrils suspended in

TABLE 7.1 Classification of amyloid

Distribution	Typical	Atypical
Primary	Rare (AA)	Common (AL)
Secondary	Infections (AA)	
	Rheumatoid Arthritis	Myeloma (AL)
Familial	FMF (AA)	Portuguese (AFp)

Typical = predominately liver, spleen and kidneys
Atypical = predominately gastrointestinal tract, heart, peripheral
           nerves and kidneys
AL   = Amyloid light chain
AFp   = Amyloid pre-albumin
AA   = Amyloid A protein

an amorphous ground substance. The material is deposited around the small vessels of many organs, but classically the liver, spleen and kidneys are most severely affected.

Primary amyloid and amyloid secondary to myeloma are due to the deposition of polymerised light chains. The organs involved include the kidney, gastrointestinal tract, peripheral nerves and the myocardium.

Familial amyloid has many different forms, the most common being familial Mediterranean fever which occurs in Sephardic Jews and gives rise to acute attacks of fever, joint pains, abdominal crises and, after several years, the nephrotic syndrome and progressive renal failure.

CLINICAL FEATURES OF RENAL AMYLOID

Renal involvement in secondary amyloid is the most serious aspect of the syndrome. Patients may present with proteinuria discovered at a medical examination or frank nephrotic syndrome. Hypertension is rarely an early feature but develops in about 50 per cent. Progress to renal failure occurs in the majority over some years, 50 per cent of the patients being dead or on dialysis within four years of diagnosis. Renal vein thrombosis is said to be a common complication and should be suspected if the patient suffers flank pain, haematuria, acceleration of renal failure or pulmonary thromboembolism.

INVESTIGATIONS

Early in the disease the kidneys are enlarged but are otherwise normal; as the disease advances, the kidneys become smaller. The diagnosis of amyloid depends upon obtaining a biopsy of affected tissue. The common biopsy sites are the kidney, rectum or gum. If the patient has had a recent operation, e.g. cholecystectomy or prostatectomy, it is worth asking for that specimen to be stained for amyloid. If no such tissue is available and the patient presents with proteinuria, then the kidney is the most rewarding organ to biopsy. It should be stained with congo red, thioflavine T or sirius red and examined by birefringent light to reveal the characteristic appearances of amyloid.

TREATMENT

Some recovery of renal function may occur if the underlying disorder can be effectively treated. Otherwise, the progress of the disease cannot be arrested and only symptomatic relief can be offered.

Obstruction

Obstructive uropathy may develop as a result of tuberculosis affecting the ureters or schistosomiasis due to *S. haematobium*. Both are rare in Britain but tuberculosis remains comparatively common in the under-developed parts of the world and *S. haematobium* infections are very common in parts of the Middle East.

Immune complex disease

Any organism, be it viral, bacterial or protozoal, may and probably does release free antigen into the circulation. The fate of that antigen depends on the patient's immune response. If antibodies are produced but in insufficient amounts to clear all the antigen, then immune complexes will circulate and a proportion will be deposited in the GBM where complement will be fixed and an inflammatory reaction ensue. Organisms which have caused immune complex nephritis are:

Bacterial
  Streptococci
  Staphylococci
  Mycobacterium leprae
  Actinobacillus
Ricketsial
  Coxiella burnetti
  Psittacosis
Viral
  Coxsackie
  Epstein–Barr virus
  Hepatitis B
  ECHO
  Guillain–Barré syndrome
Parasitic
  P. malariae
  Schistosoma mansoni
  Toxoplasma gondii

The role of streptococci has already been discussed. The following are two examples of nephropathies associated with infections.

MALARIAL NEPHROPATHY

This is perhaps the most common identified cause of immune complex renal disease in the world. It is only associated with *Plasmodium malariae* infection, and where this has been eradicated, a dramatic decline in the incidence of glomerular diseases in that area has followed, as was carefully documented in British Guiana. Patients present with proteinuria, the nephrotic syndrome or renal failure. Their serum complement remains normal throughout the course of the illness. Spontaneous remissions are common, but so is progression to terminal renal failure and rather surprisingly anti-malarial therapy does not appear to influence the course of the disease.

SUB-ACUTE INFECTIVE ENDOCARDITIS

This is one of the most common identified infections which gives rise to chronic immune complex nephritis in Britain. Not every patient who suffers from endocarditis develops clinical evidence of renal disease. Men are more often affected than women. The most common manifestations are haematuria and proteinuria; the nephrotic syndrome is rare, but renal failure does occur and progresses until the infection has been eradicated. Renal involvement is associated with hypocomplementaemia. Therefore, any patient with a valvular disease, proteinuria and a low concentration of C4 or C3 in the blood, should be assumed to have endocarditis even if they feel well and are afebrile. Effective treatment will restore the complement levels to normal and improve renal function. The C4 concentration is a good guide both to the efficacy of treatment and to reactivation of infection.

MALIGNANCY AND THE RENAL TRACT

Tumours may arise within the kidney and urinary tract, and the clinical consequences will be discussed in Chapters 15 and 17. Clinically important metastases to the kidney are surprisingly rare in view of the very high blood flow. However, tumours arising elsewhere may affect the kidney in other ways.

Obstruction

This is caused by tumours of the bladder, prostate and cervix which have spread to involve both ureters. Treatment is rarely effective except in patients with carcinoma of the prostate. Retroperitoneal tumours may encase the ureters, so that the calyces become dilated but do not obstruct the passage of retrograde catheters. Surgical relief may be obtained by diverting the ureters into an ileal loop.

Hypercalcaemia

The common causes of a serum calcium greater than 3 mmol/l are parathyroid tumour or hyperplasia, a carcinoma of another organ (particularly the bronchus) which produces parathormone ectopically or multiple bony metastases. Severe hypercalcaemia is often associated with acute renal failure. Serum calcium may be lowered by rehydration of the patient with saline combined with calcitonin, mithramycin or neutral phosphate given intravenously.

Steroids are usually ineffective. The definitive treatment requires removal of the tumour.

Hyperuricaemia

Abrupt rises in the serum concentration of urate may cause renal failure due to super-saturation of the urine leading to tubular deposition and intra-renal obstruction. This happens most commonly when there is a massive cellular breakdown during the early stages of treatment of acute myeloproliferative disorders. For this reason, allopurinol (300 mg/day), a xanthine oxidase inhibitor should be included in the treatment regime. Urate deposition may be minimised by alkalinsing the urine and ensuring a urine volume of 3 1/24 hours. If renal failure is already established, the patient should be dialysed. Spontaneous resolution usually occurs after serum urate has returned to normal.

Glomerulopathies

Immune complexes are demonstrable in the serum of the majority of patients with any type of carcinoma. Clinically important renal disease mediated by immune complexes is much rarer. Patients usually present with the nephrotic syndrome and a normal creatinine clearance. The changes of membranous nephropathy are found on renal biopsy and indeed ten per cent of patients with this pathological diagnosis are subsequently discovered to have a tumour. Successful removal of the tumour is followed by remission of the nephrotic syndrome but this is unfortunately rare.

Hodgkin's disease and occasionally other forms of lymphoma are associated with the nephrotic syndrome due to minimal change nephropathy. These patients do not respond to steroids in the normal manner, but remissions occur when the lymphoma is effectively treated. Recurrences may be detected by the reappearance of proteinuria.

Amyloid

Some tumours, particularly myeloma, may promote the deposition of amyloid in the kidney causing proteinuria or the nephrotic syndrome. This is rare.

DIABETES MELLITUS

Diabetes mellitus is the most common metabolic disease which affects the kidneys and the likelihood of developing clinically important disease increases the longer the patient has been diabetic. Only six per cent of all diabetics die of renal failure, but this increases to 50 per cent among those patients who develop diabetes before the age of ten. Many more have significant renal abnormalities at the time of death. There are several ways in which diabetes can affect the kidneys.

Acute diabetic ketoacidosis

Patients present with gross dehydration, hyperglycaemia and acidosis. Renal failure is surprisingly rare in view of the degree of dehydration. Perhaps the diuresis induced by the glycosuria may help to protect the kidney.

Urinary tract infection

Diabetic patients who have no urinary tract abnormality are no more prone to urinary tract infections than non-diabetics but the clinical consequences are likely to be more severe in the diabetic. In particular, acute pyelonephritis develops more commonly. Therefore, infections should be detected as early as possible and treated vigorously.

Papillary necrosis

Acute pyelonephritis in an elderly diabetic may lead to papillary necrosis (see Chapter 4).

Neurogenic bladder

Patients who have been diabetic for more than ten years may develop a diabetic neuropathy affecting the autonomic nervous system. Bladder involvement may give rise to poor urinary stream, increased frequency, post-micturition dribbling and incomplete emptying of the bladder. This may accelerate the development of the renal failure and increase the liability to infection. Catheterisation should be avoided, if possible. Manual expression of the bladder, resection of the bladder neck, and parasympathomimetic drugs may help.

Diabetic glomerular disease

This is the most important renal complication of diabetes. It causes proteinuria often of sufficient magnitude to lead to the nephrotic syndrome, hypertension and progressive renal failure. Proteinuria usully develops 10–15 years after the onset of insulin dependent and independent diabetes. It is a more common cause of death among the former because elderly diabetics often die of major vessel disease. The rapidity of decline of renal function is proportional to the amount of proteinuria. Most patients will also have diabetic retinopathy which testifies to the diffuse nature of the vascular disease.

PATHOLOGY

The specific lesions of diabetic glomerulopathy are (a) nodules of hyaline-like material found in the capillary loops and mesangium, originally described by Kimmelstiel and Wilson in 1936 and (b) capsular drops which are tear-shaped accumulations of eosinophilic material in Bowman's capsule (Fig. 7.2). Not all patients have these lesions. The most common abnormality is *diffuse glomerular sclerosis* which is found in 75 per cent of biopsies. This consists of PAS-positive material found in the mesangium and the glomerular basement membrane. The walls of the capillary loops become progressively thickened until the lumena are obliterated.

TREATMENT

No effective treatment exists. Good diabetic control may retard the progress of diabetic nephropathy, although many patients with apparently excellent control over many years still develop renal failure. Hypophysectomy may reduce the severity of glomerular lesions, but it is contraindicated in patients with reduced renal function, as further deterioration occurs after the operation, presumably because of the absence of growth hormone. Dialysis and renal transplantation are being used to treat an increasing number of diabetics with terminal renal failure but are not as

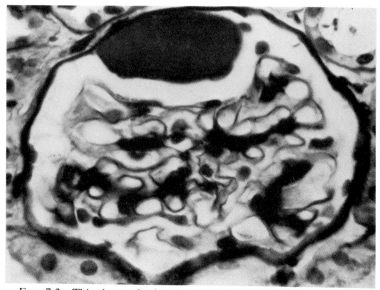

FIG. 7.2 This glomerulus in a kidney of a diabetic patient contains a capsular drop.

successful as in non-diabetics, although survival is now as high as 40 per cent over three years.

POINTS OF EMPHASIS

● Renal biopsy should be performed in patients with SLE who have proteinuria, nephrotic syndrome or deteriorating renal function.

● Steroids in high doses should be given to patients with diffuse lupus nephritis and the dose titrated against renal function.

● The finding of a focal proliferative or crescentic nephritis, without diffuse deposits of immunoglobulin, in a patient with multi-organ disease, is sufficiently suggestive of PAN to justify a trial of steroids.

● The development of proteinuria in rheumatoid disease suggests either a drug-induced side-effect or the development of amyloidosis.

● Rheumatoid arthritis and chronic infection, particularly tuberculosis, are the commonest causes of secondary amyloidosis.

● Renal involvement is the most serious aspect of secondary amyloidosis.

● Malarial nephropathy is a common cause of immune complex renal disease.

● Patients with valvular heart disease, proteinuria or haematuria, and hypocomplementaemia, should be thoroughly investigated for infective endocarditis even if they feel well.

● Although metastases to the kidney are rare, malignant disease may affect renal function by causing urinary obstruction, immune complex disease, amyloidosis, hypercalcaemia or hyperuricaemia.

● The acute development of hyperuricaemia may cause acute renal failure. Its occurrence during the early treatment of myeloproliferative disorders can be prevented by the addition of allopurinol 300 mg/day to the treatment regime.

● Fifty per cent of patients who develop diabetes before the age of ten die of renal failure.

● Good diabetic control may retard the progress of diabetic nephropathy.

CHAPTER 8

Diseases of the renal vasculature

INFARCTION OF THE KIDNEY

This usually results either from arterial thrombosis or from an embolus; the latter is much more common. Bilateral occlusion can occur but is rare. Thrombosis usually occurs as a consequence of atheroma of the artery and may be superimposed on a stenosis or follow trauma. An embolus may arise from an atheromatous aorta, the left atrium, a left ventricular mural thrombus or in bacterial endocarditis.

Diagnosis

The classical description is of severe loin pain often accompanied by vomiting with fever, loin tenderness and haematuria, usually microscopic only, on urine examination. Hypertension often follows after a few days and may be persistent or transient. This clinical picture is by no means invariable, and probably in at least 50 per cent of cases the occurrence of infarction goes unrecognized. An IVU shortly after the infarct will show absent or markedly reduced dye excretion. As this appearance is non-specific, other causes of unilateral absence or impairment of renal function such as ureteric obstruction may have to be excluded by retrograde pyelography. In infarction, a normal calyceal pattern will be seen. By three weeks, a repeat IVU will usually demonstrate symmetrical shrinkage of the kidney. Serum enzyme measurement may help in the diagnosis with a rise of lactic dehydrogenase (LDH) from about the second to fourteenth day and glutamic oxalacetic transaminase (GOT) for a few days only. Traumatic rupture of the renal artery may be caused by a blow to the back. Other injuries are usually present as well as extensive bruising. Aortography is the quickest way of making the diagnosis.

Management

While it is often assumed that surgical intervention is unlikely to be successful, some surgeons have reported recovery of renal function with immediate thrombectomy. Thus, if the patient is not too ill or old, exploration of the kidney may be indicated. Persistent, severe hypertension following unilateral infarction is rare but, when present, is an indication for nephrectomy. Nephrectomy or arterial repair may be required following traumatic rupture of the renal artery.

RENAL VEIN THROMBOSIS

This may cause infarction in infancy where it occurs as a complication of dehydration. In the adult it is usually either a consequence of thrombosis of the inferior vena cava or arises in conjunction with renal amyloid or glomerulonephritis. Although the nephrotic syndrome is a common accompaniment of renal vein thrombosis, it is probably due to the associated glomerular lesion rather than the thrombosis. Unlike the condition in childhood, infarction rarely complicates renal vein thrombosis in the adult.

RENOVASCULAR HYPERTENSION

This term is defined as potentially remediable hypertension of renal origin to distinguish it from the hypertension of chronic parenchymal renal disease which is treatable but not curable.

Renal artery stenosis (RAS)

Although by far the most common of the renovascular causes, this condition only accounts for a few per cent of an unselected group of hypertensive patients. The pathological basis is either atheroma which is responsible for two-thirds or fibromuscular dysplasia (or hyperplasia) in the remaining one-third of patients. The disease is most common in the middle-aged and elderly and in this age group atheroma is almost always the cause. Fibromuscular dysplasia is a disease of unknown aetiology in which there is thickening of the media of the arterial wall often causing a long stenotic segment or multiple areas of stenosis. The female to male sex ratio is 4:1 and it usually affects young adults.

DIAGNOSIS

There are no reliable clinical leads to help distinguish RAS from idiopathic (essential) hypertension. Having said this, there are a few points which occur more commonly in RAS, namely an abdominal bruit (in about 40 per cent), hypertension in the malignant phase, and age below 35 years. The decision as to who should be screened for RAS is controversial. A reasonable policy is to screen all who are young or have malignant phase hypertension or any other clinical pointer. Screening should consist of an IVU of the following type. There should be rapid sequence films at the beginning, e.g. at one minute intervals up to five minutes, and a water load at 15–20 minutes with a further one or two films thereafter. The abnormalities which may be seen on the affected side are:

Reduced kidney size.
Delayed appearance of pyelogram.
Spastic appearance of calyces.
Delayed excretion of dye in the later films despite a water load.
Indentations in upper ureter (due to collateral blood vessels).

These features are, of course, mainly observed in comparison with the normal side and are therefore worthless in the occasional patient with bilateral stenosis. Where there is an abnormal IVU or strong clinical suspicion, the next step is an arteriogram. The demonstration of a stenosis by arteriography does not prove that it is the cause of the hypertension as more than 50 per cent occlusion of the artery is required to affect renal blood flow. Although an abnormal IVU is strongly suggestive of a functionally active stenosis, further investigation is usually performed. There are three techniques available, isotope renography, measurement of renin in renal vein blood samples and divided renal function studies. This last technique involves bilateral ureteric catheterisation with measurement of urine volume and sodium concentration and renal blood flow for each kidney.

MANAGEMENT

Until recently surgery was preferred in the young patient or in severe hypertension. The choice of technique lies among some form of arterial reconstruction, a bypass graft and nephrectomy. Two developments are currently reducing the indications for surgery. One is the introduction of percutaneous transluminal angioplasty. This technique consists of dilatation of the stenosis with a balloon catheter under arteriographic control. The other development is the introduction of more potent antihypertensive drugs, in particular those which specifically inhibit the renin–angiotensin system, of which captopril is one of the first examples.

Other renovascular causes

Rarely, other arterial abnormalities can be present such as an aneurysm, or narrowing due to extrinsic pressure, e.g. from a tumour. More common is unilateral parenchymal renal disease usually due to pyelonephritis and rarely to tuberculosis or other cause. The main aid to diagnosis is the IVU. Surgical treatment consists of nephrectomy but a good blood pressure response is seen in only about one-third of patients and therefore operation is indicated only if the patient is young, the hypertension poorly controlled by drugs and the other kidney is unequivocally normal on X-ray.

ESSENTIAL HYPERTENSION

There is no single cause for this disease. It is even argued whether it is a disease or simply one end of the blood pressure spectrum in the population. The aetiological factors include heredity, body sodium content, the renin–angiotensin system and the sympathetic nervous system.

Types

Subdivision is according to the severity, the two grades being benign and malignant. The latter occurs in only about 5 per cent of patients with essential hypertension in contrast to a much higher percentage, around 15–20 per cent, in hypertension secondary to renal disease. The criterion of the malignant phase is based on its effect on small blood vessels as judged by fundal examination. Haemorrhages, exudates and papilloedema are the three features looked for, any one of which indicates the malignant phase. The blood pressure reading itself does not differentiate the two types and severe, long-standing hypertension is frequently benign.

Diagnosis

Essential hypertension is diagnosed by exclusion of the renal, endocrine and cardiovascular causes. There are no features which are specific for the essential type although a family history is a clinical pointer.

Effect on renal structure

Benign hypertension, even of long standing, may have little effect on the renal vessels. The changes which are seen include reduplication of the internal elastic lamina in the larger vessels and deposition of hyaline material in the wall of arterioles. By contrast, in malignant hypertension severe vessel damage occurs, the main lesion being intimal proliferation with, less often, fibrinoid necrosis of small arteries and arterioles. Renal function usually deteriorates so rapidly that there is insufficient time for shrinkage of the kidney before presentation. Thus a relatively normal bipolar length is seen on X-ray in renal failure due to essential but malignant hypertension which contrasts with the small kidneys seen in chronic glomerulonephritis and chronic pyelonephritis.

Effect on renal function

In parallel with the structural changes, benign hypertension is associated with little or no functional abnormality while the malignant phase results in rapid deterioration of renal function.

Transition from benign to malignant phase

There is good evidence that localised intravascular coagulation in the small renal vessels has an important role in the transition. The deposition of platelets and their release of enzymes and vasoactive agents initiates a vicious circle which results in further thrombus formation. Another effect of this chain of events is the development of microangiopathic haemolytic anaemia (see below). The most important point, the initial triggering factor to this chain of events, is still not clear.

Management

The most controversial decision is who to treat. There is now general agreement that asymptomatic hypertension justifies therapy in some cases. A reasonable policy would be to treat a young adult with a resting diastolic blood pressure consistently greater than 95 mmHg. The comparable figure in the 40–60 age range would be 105 mm Hg while above 60 years there has to be a flexible policy. First line therapy consists of a beta blocker and/or diuretics (see Table 10.5, page 195). If control is poor, a vasodilator such as hydralazine or prazosin can be added. The newer vasodilator drug minoxidil is extremely potent but regularly produces hirsutism so is less suitable for females, and also has to be given with frusemide to combat sodium retention. Drugs acting centrally are less useful, and of this group, clonidine is preferred to methyldopa.

Finally, the most exciting area of therapy relates to antagonists of the renin–angiotensin system (e.g. captopril) although their role in essential hypertension, in which renin is not an obvious primary factor, is not yet clear.

THROMBOTIC MICROANGIOPATHY

This condition consists of the widespread formation of thrombi in small blood vessels leading to ischaemic necrosis of the organ. While it may involve a number of organs, the renal vasculature is almost always affected, and may lead to acute renal failure.

Pathogenesis

A number of diseases can trigger the formation of intravascular fibrin thrombi. The deposition of these in the small arteries and arterioles of the kidney leads to a variable degree of ischaemic necrosis. In addition, the uneven and irregular deposition of fibrin thrombi causes trauma to the red blood cells in their passage through the small vessels. This produces fragmentation of the cells which can be seen on a blood film and the end result is micro-angiopathic haemolytic anaemia. Finally, the incorporation of platelets, fibrin and other clotting factors in the thrombi impairs the blood coagulation mechanism leading to a bleeding tendency. The full blown syndrome is entitled disseminated intravascular coagulation (DIC). The term thrombotic microangiopathy describes the pathology within the blood vessels and if this is extensive it may be associated with the clinical syndrome of DIC with its widespread effects.

Effect on renal function

This is variable, but widespread intravascular coagulation can lead to extensive cortical necrosis. Unlike acute tubular necrosis, this is an irreversible lesion and a proportion of or even all renal function will be permanently lost depending on the extent of the necrosis.

Causes

Although the association with the following disorders is well established, the mechanism by which the intravascular thrombosis is initiated is not well understood.

OBSTETRIC COMPLICATIONS

Pre-eclampsia

This condition consists of proteinuria, hypertension and oedema usually occurring after the 28th week of pregnancy but occasionally earlier. In extreme cases, it can lead to eclampsia with convulsions, cardiac failure and renal failure. Also it increases fetal mortality with a high incidence of intrauterine death and prematurity. Intravascular thrombosis may well not be the prime cause of pre-eclampsia although it is a constant feature. Uncomplicated pre-eclampsia does not cause more than mild impairment of renal function but cortical necrosis may follow the development of eclampsia.

Post-partum renal failure

In this unusual condition acute renal failure due to cortical necrosis occurs a few days to a few weeks after the end of what may have been an entirely normal pregnancy. The cortical necrosis is usually extensive or even complete so that renal function may not recover. The trigger mechanism for the intravascular thrombosis is unknown.

Other obstetric causes

Septic abortion, concealed accidental haemorrhage and amniotic fluid embolism may all be complicated by acute renal failure which may recover only partly because of a variable degree of cortical necrosis.

HAEMATOLOGICAL DISORDERS

Haemolytic uraemic syndrome

The typical picture is the onset of a febrile illness in an infant or young child, often with diarrhoea and vomiting and followed by miocroangiopathic haemolytic anaemia and acute renal failure. A bacterial or other pathogen may be the triggering factor but proof is lacking. Progressive chronic renal failure may develop despite recovery of renal function in the short term but full recovery is the rule under the age of four years.

Thrombotic thrombocytopenic purpura (TTP)

The usual features are microangiopathic haemolytic anaemia, thrombocytopenic purpura, acute renal failure, fluctuating neurological signs and fever. This condition has often been said to be the adult equivalent of the haemolytic uraemic syndrome and it carries a high mortality. It was first described long before the concept of DIC was established and it is fairly certain that these two conditions are the same. In other words, the name TTP has been used in the past to describe cases of DIC in which no obvious triggering illness was apparent.

Other haematological disorders which can cause thrombotic

microangiopathy include acute leukaemia and the crises of sickle cell anaemia.

INFECTIONS

Although bacteraemia due to Gram-negative bacilli is the most common, other bacterial and also probably viral and rickettsial infections can cause intravascular coagulation. Cortical necrosis is a rare sequel although acute tubular necrosis, which is fully recoverable, is a well-recognised complication.

RENAL DISORDERS

Two conditions which arise within the kidney and may cause thrombotic microangiopathy are rapidly progressive glomerulonephritis and transplant rejection. In neither is the thrombosis usually extensive enough to cause a major degree of DIC.

Management

In addition to specific treatment of the disease which is causing the thrombotic microangiopathy, there is sometimes a case for anticoagulant therapy. This is usually given in the form of heparin and the two main aims are to correct the coagulation defect resulting from the DIC and to prevent renal cortical necrosis. This latter aim may not be achieved especially if the onset of treatment is delayed. Also it may require courage to prescribe heparin for a patient with a serious coagulation defect but it is undoubtedly beneficial in some patients. The prognosis is poor with regard to both survival of the patient and recovery of renal function.

VASCULAR INVOLVEMENT IN MULTISYSTEM DISEASE

The important diseases in this category include polyarteritis, scleroderma, SLE, Henoch–Schonlein syndrome and diabetes mellitus. All are dealt with in Chapter 7 and will therefore not be discussed here.

POINTS OF EMPHASIS

- Renal infarction is usually due to an arterial embolus.

- Patients with malignant hypertension, an abdominal bruit or under the age of 35 should be screened for RAS.

- RAS caused by fibromuscular dysplasia usually affects young women.

- The development of more effective hypotensive drugs and of the technique of percutaneous transluminal angioplasty are reducing the indications for surgery in RAS.

- Malignant hypertension develops in only five per cent of subjects with essential hypertension but in 15–20 per cent of patients with hypertension secondary to renal disease.

- Long-standing benign hypertension may have little effect on renal vessels.

- Severe renal vessel damage occurs in malignant hypertension producing a rapid deterioration in renal function.

- Thrombotic microangiopathy almost always affects the renal vasculature and may cause ARF.

- Severe thrombotic microangiopathy may result in DIC which can lead to irreversible cortical necrosis.

- Heparin therapy may be indicated in thrombotic microangiopathy.

CHAPTER 9

Acute renal failure

INTRODUCTION

Acute renal failure (ARF) can only be defined in very broad terms, namely 'renal failure of sudden onset'. An early priority is accurate diagnosis and the first step is the differentiation of acute from chronic renal failure (CRF). Attention is usually first drawn to the possibility of ARF by the finding of oliguria or a high blood urea. If the onset of the renal failure occurs in hospital, a previous normal blood urea will make the differentiation from CRF. Without this guide, other points may help. The best pointer to ARF is the recent onset of a serious illness in a previously healthy person. The presence of CRF is suggested by the slow progression of such symptoms as tiredness, dyspnoea, nocturia and anorexia and the findings of hypertension and severe anaemia. If small kidneys can be demonstrated by an abdominal X-ray or IVU, this will clinch the diagnosis of CRF but normal renal size does not necessarily mean that the renal failure is acute. There may of course be a combination of the two, that is 'acute on chronic' renal failure and this is discussed in Chapter 10. The differentiation of ARF from CRF is followed by an attempt to delineate the type of ARF. The elementary mistake of confusing oliguria with acute retention must be avoided by confirming that the bladder is empty and this nearly always requires catheterisation. ARF itself can be of three types, pre-renal, obstructive, and that due to intrinsic renal damage. These three types will now be considered individually including the assessment required to distinguish between them.

PRE-RENAL TYPE

A sudden reduction in blood volume for any reason will result in a reduced renal blood flow. As a consequence, the glomerular filtration rate falls leading to reduced solute excretion. At the same time, there is stimulation of antidiuretic hormone and aldosterone production resulting in oliguria with a concentrated urine and sometimes a rise in blood urea. This is the pre-renal or functional type of ARF. If the reduction of blood volume (oligaemia) remains uncorrected for several hours or longer, renal vasoconstriction will develop, leading to ischaemia and acute tubular necrosis (ATN). The pathogenesis of this will be discussed later in the chapter. Thus the pre-renal type and ATN share a common basic cause, the main difference being in the severity and duration of the insult. In contrast to ATN, the pre-renal type is a transient phenomenon which often goes unnoticed prior to and during the resuscitation of a shocked patient and it should resolve as the blood volume is restored to normal. Management is directed at the patient's circulation and not at the kidney.

OBSTRUCTIVE ACUTE RENAL FAILURE

AETIOLOGY

Acute obstruction is usually due to either a ureteric calculus in a patient with a solitary kidney or a malignant tumour involving both ureters. The tumours most often encountered are carcinoma of the cervix or body of the uterus, of the bladder, prostate or rectum, or metastases in lymph nodes in the posterior abdominal wall. The usual mechanism is that the tumour first obstructs one ureter leading to non-function of the kidney but without producing symptoms. Later, when the tumour spreads to obstruct the other ureter, the patient presents with sudden onset of anuria. Occasionally retroperitoneal fibrosis may cause obstruction of acute onset although often it will present in a more insidious manner.

PRESENTATION

Obstruction is the cause of ARF in only a small percentage of cases but it is important to exclude the possibility in the presence of a suggestive presentation. A patient with a solitary kidney or history of calculous disease is one such presentation. Another is the existence of a tumour, particularly arising in the pelvis, usually from the uterus or bladder. Thus ARF with vaginal bleeding in the older female or profuse haematuria are suggestive. Clinical features resulting from the obstruction itself are inconstant. Loin pain is relatively infrequent although loin tenderness and a palpable kidney are common. Anuria rather than the oliguria typical of ATN is a useful hint. However, anuria is also typical of rapidly progressive glomerulonephritis (see below) or the rare problem of arterial thrombosis. Finally absence of the type of preceding acute illness that leads to ATN (see below) should raise the suspicion of obstruction.

INVESTIGATION

The intravenous urogram (IVU) should usually be the first investigation undertaken. A high dose of contrast medium (up to 2·2 ml/kg of Hypaque 45 per cent or equivalent) and tomography are both essential and the patient should not be dehydrated. The abnormalities which may indicate obstruction are:

Calculus
Asymmetry of kidney size
Increasing density of nephrogram
Negative shadow
Delayed pyelogram
Dilated ureter

A calculus in the pelvis or ureter will confirm the diagnosis provided the opposite kidney is absent or non-functioning. Asymmetry of renal size is often best seen on the tomogram films and the most frequent finding is enlargement of the obstructed kidney often with shrinkage on the opposite side due to long-standing damage. A delay in appearance of the nephrogram with progressive increase in density is indicative of obstruction and therefore late films, the last one at 24 hours, are important. By contrast, in acute tubular necrosis the nephrogram appears early and persists but does not progressively increase in density and is not followed by a pyelogram. The negative shadow sometimes seen in an obstructed kidney consists of a rim of opacified parenchyma surrounding dilated but not yet opacified calyces and pelvis and this may be followed by the late appearance of a pyelogram. Good technique is essential to demonstrate all these features. Once the IVU has shown which kidney is obstructed, a retrograde or antegrade pyelogram is required to delineate the site and nature of the obstruction.

Ultrasound is being used with increasing success to diagnose obstruction in the presence of renal failure. Images show dilated calyces and pelvis and may even give information on the site and cause of obstruction since cysts, stones, tumours and retroperitoneal fibrosis all have distinct images.

Retrograde ureteric catheterisation is carried out at the same time as cystoscopy, the latter being necessary to exclude a bladder tumour, and an ascending ureterogram can then be performed. It may be possible to pass the catheter beyond the obstruction and it can then be left *in situ* to effect temporary drainage. Obstruction due to retroperitoneal fibrosis or tumour will not usually occlude the lumen of the ureter but causes obstruction by infiltration of the muscle layer and inhibition of peristalsis. Thus free passage of the catheter up the ureter does not rule out an obstructive cause.

The antegrade pyelogram is a recently introduced alternative to the retrograde method. This technique involves percutaneous puncture of the dilated calyceal system with a needle; localisation is probably best provided by ultrasound. Dye can then be injected directly into the pelvi-calyceal system.

Isotope renography can confirm the presence of ureteric obstruction but gives no information on the nature or site of the obstruction and is therefore of limited value.

MANAGEMENT

If free drainage cannot be achieved through a ureteric catheter, a nephrostomy is carried out with the insertion of a drain into the renal pelvis through a loin incision or by a catheter inserted by direct puncture of a dilated calyx under ultrasound or X-ray control. This will permit return of renal function and thereafter the indications for, and type of, definitive surgery will depend on the underlying pathology. Relief of the obstruction is a matter of urgency but once drainage has been established, definitive surgery is often best delayed for one or two weeks or longer to allow time for improvement in the patient's fitness. In some cases of advanced metastatic tumour, surgery may not be indicated at all, as death from uraemia might be preferable to death from other manifestations of metastatic disease.

INTRINSIC RENAL DISEASE

The diseases which may produce ARF by damage to the kidneys themselves are:

Acute tubular necrosis
  Ischaemic
  Toxic

Miscellaneous
  Rapidly progressive glomerulonephritis (Chapter 6)
  Vasculitis (Chapter 7)
  Malignant hypertension (Chapter 8)
  Papillary necrosis (Chapter 4)
  Hepatorenal syndrome
  Intravascular coagulation (Chapter 8)
  Acute interstitial nephritis (Chapter 4)
  Intratubular obstruction
  Severe hypercalcaemia

Thrombosis
  Arterial
  Venous

Apart from acute tubular necrosis (ATN), all are either uncommon or rare.

Acute tubular necrosis

Two mechanisms can produce ATN, ischaemia which accounts for more than 80 per cent of cases, and toxins which are responsible for the remainder. The aetiology of the two types will be considered separately although in some patients both mechanisms are involved.

AETIOLOGY

Ischaemic type

The prime factor in almost all cases is a reduction in effective blood volume (oligaemia) leading to a marked fall in renal blood flow and to a very low glomerular filtration rate (GFR). This is the main reason for the oliguria rather than any tubular damage. There were two previous hypotheses of which the first suggested that passive back diffusion of glomerular filtrate through necrotic tubular epithelial cells into the peritubular capillaries resulted in the oliguria. The second proposed that debris in the tubular lumen caused intrarenal obstruction. Both these ideas can now be dismissed as irrelevant. The main controversy today relates to the mechanism by which the lowered renal blood flow causes such a profound fall in GFR and the reason why the urine volume may remain low for several weeks after restoration of the blood flow. Two mechanisms have been recognised as probably important. The first is the renin-angiotensin system. Oligaemia and reduced renal blood flow cause renin release and the resultant renal vasoconstriction may lead to the setting up of a vicious circle. High plasma renin and angiotensin levels in ATN are well documented, although this does not prove a cause and effect relationship. The second mechanism of probable relevance is swelling of the endothelial cells lining the glomerular capillaries. This has been demonstrated by electron microscopy and will impede glomerular filtration.

Of more practical importance than the above theories of pathogenesis are the clinical settings in which ATN is likely to occur. These can be summarised as any cause of hypotension, oligaemia or reduced renal perfusion if of sufficient duration and severity, particularly in patients predisposed by such things as old age or sodium depletion. The predisposing diseases most often seen in clinical practice are listed in Table 9.1. The surgical group usually accounts for about 65 per cent, the medical group 30 per cent, and the obstetric group around 5 per cent.

Nephrotoxic type

The mechanism of damage is not clear although there are good reasons why the kidney is particularly susceptible to toxicity. Such

TABLE 9.1   Causes of ischaemic type of acute tubular necrosis.

Surgical	Medical	Obstetric
Multiple injuries	Bacteraemia	Abortion
Perforated peptic ulcer	Pneumonia	Ante-partum haemorrhage
Gastro-intestinal haemorrhage	Gastroenteritis	Post-partum haemorrhage
Pancreatitis	Severe fluid and electrolyte depletion	
Biliary tract infection	Myocardial infarct	
Ruptured aortic aneurysm		
Cardiac surgery		
Burns		

reasons include the high renal blood flow, the permeable endothelial lining of the capillaries and the very high concentration of solutes which may be achieved in the medulla. Some of the known nephrotoxins are as follows:

Drugs
　Antibiotics
　　Aminoglycosides (gentamicin, kanamycin, neomycin, amikacin, tobramycin, streptomycin)
　　Cephaloridine (and some other cephalosporins)
　　Tetracycline
　Others
　　Paracetamol overdose
　　Sulphonamides
　　Amphotericin B
Pigments
　Intravascular haemolysis (infections, e.g. malaria, septicaemia; drugs and chemicals; mismatched blood transfusion)
　Myoglobinuria (crush injury, barbiturate poisoning, alcohol withdrawal, convulsions, hyperosmolar coma and coxsackie B infection)
Metals
　Mercury
　Bismuth
　Copper

Solvents
  Carbon tetrachloride
  Ethylene glycol
  Trichlorethylene
Miscellaneous
  Chlorates
  Paraquat
  Snake venom
  Mushrooms
  Phenol
  Quinine

Those of most importance are drugs and in particular antibiotics. Of these, gentamicin is probably the most widely used as it is usually highly effective. Nephrotoxicity is more common with high serum levels but can occur with therapeutic levels and it is not clear whether high peak or high trough levels are more dangerous. Cephaloridine and tetracycline should be avoided in high risk patients such as those with pre-existing impairment of renal function. Both free haemoglobin and myoglobin can, in high concentration, result in ATN and examples of predisposing causes are mentioned above. Two fairly common toxins are paracetamol when taken in overdose and paraquat. Although in the case of these two substances the liver and lung damage respectively are often the main manifestations, ATN is common. Most other nephrotoxins are rarities.

DIAGNOSIS

ATN has to be differentiated from other intrinsic renal diseases and from the pre-renal type. The most characteristic point about ATN is the preceding acute incident which is usually associated with features such as hypotension, blood loss or high fever. However, the acute incident may not be so readily apparent, particularly in the elderly. In the few cases where differentiation from some other intrinsic renal disease cannot be made on clinical grounds, renal biopsy will be required. A much more common need is to distinguish between ATN and the pre-renal type. They have a common pathogenesis, the main difference being in the duration and degree of the precipitating incident. Thus patients who become oligaemic enter the pre-renal stage and if the oligaemia cannot be corrected fairly rapidly, they pass through to the stage of established ATN. Differentiation of these two causes of oliguria can be made in two ways. Firstly, restoration of blood volume and cardiac output will produce a diuresis in the pre-renal type but not in ATN. Secondly the urine concentration will distinguish the two stages and show too the intermediate stage, so-called incipient ATN. The figures shown in Table 9.2 cannot be applied rigidly but are only intended as a guide. The use of osmolality measurement carries more precision than urea, and expression of the results as a urine/plasma ratio is more meaningful than the use of urine measurements alone.

TABLE 9.2 Differential diagnosis of oliguria.

	Urine/plasma osmolality ratio	Urine/plasma urea ratio
Pre-renal	>1·7:1	>14:1
Incipient acute tubular necrosis	17·1:1 to 1·1:1	14:1 to 5:1
Established acute tubular necrosis	<1·1:1	<5:1

CLINICAL COURSE

This is divided into oliguric, diuretic and recovery phases.

Oliguric phase

Oliguria is a common but not invariable feature of ATN. In a few patients, a dilute urine of normal volume is accompanied by a rising blood urea. However, in most cases the volume varies from a few ml to 100–200 ml per day. The mean duration of this phase is ten days but the range is wide, from 1 to about 50 days. The development of fluid overload can easily occur even with fairly careful control of intake, so oedema, a raised jugular venous pressure and pulmonary crepitations may occur. The blood pressure usually remains normal. With good management, advanced uraemia with its attendant complications (see below) should not develop, but some uraemic features may occur such as anorexia, nausea and vomiting. More important, both wound healing and resistance to infection are markedly depressed despite good control of the uraemia. In most patients, all these clinical consequences of renal failure are overshadowed by the features of the illness which caused the ATN. Almost invariably this will have produced a serious illness to which the renal failure is added.

During the oliguric phase, daily biochemical and haematological monitoring is necessary as the blood levels of urea and creatinine will usually rise fairly rapidly, especially in hypercatabolic situations such as severe infection. The serum sodium will fall if the blood volume expands with fluid overload, but the most important electrolyte abnormality is hyperkalaemia. The two main mechanisms are metabolic acidosis which favours the movement of H^+ into cells in exchange for potassium and the leakage of potassium from cells damaged by infection or trauma. Hyperkalaemia will therefore occur even with restriction of potassium intake. The haemoglobin will show a steady fall due to marrow depression and haemolysis in addition to any blood loss which may occur.

Diuretic phase

A steady rise in urine volume indicates that renal function is beginning to recover but the GFR usually rises slowly and more than a week may pass from the onset of diuresis before a spontaneous fall in blood urea occurs. The term 'diuretic' is used by convention but a rise in urine volume to well above the normal range will only occur if the patient has developed fluid overload during the oliguric phase. Serious complications and death may still occur at this stage and careful management remains essential.

Recovery phase

Renal function slowly returns towards normal over a period of weeks accompanied by restoration of well-being.

EARLY MANAGEMENT

Once the patient has established ATN, the time taken for renal function to recover cannot be influenced by any therapeutic measures. If, however, oliguria is recognised early, appropriate measures may avoid the development of established ATN. If still in the pre-renal stage, restoration of a normal blood volume and renal perfusion should produce a diuresis. Beyond this, the renal failure progresses through the incipient to the established stage of ATN over a variable period, usually some hours. There is evidence that during this incipient stage, the intravenous administration of a diuretic, either mannitol (20 g) or high dose frusemide (250–500 mg) can sometimes establish a diuresis. Dopamine may also be of value in this situation due to its effect of increasing renal blood flow. Only a low dose should be used, 2–5 μg/kg/min, unless the patient is in a state of shock, when the inotropic effect of a higher dose will be beneficial. Should oliguria persist despite correction of oligaemia and the use of these measures, it has to be accepted that the patient has established ATN.

CONSERVATIVE THERAPY OF ESTABLISHED ATN

Fluid balance

Careful monitoring of fluid balance is essential. The best method is daily weighing and this should be done whenever possible. Also accurate fluid charts should be kept at all times. Other guides are clinical examination, which is insensitive, measurement of the central venous pressure, and the use of the chest X-ray to show if there is pulmonary oedema. There is no standard guide to fluid intake. It ranges from 500 to 1500 ml per day *in excess of measurable losses*, these including urine and fluid from the gastrointestinal tract. This range in intake reflects variation in insensible fluid loss from the skin and in the expired air which increases with such things as fever, a warm environment and tachypnoea. To provide adequate nutrition, a high fluid intake is usually necessary. Ultrafiltration can be used in patients requiring dialysis to compensate for the extra fluid given (see below).

Electrolyte balance

In the absence of a large loss of gastrointestinal fluid, electrolyte loss is minimal in the oliguric patient. The two electrolytes of most importance are sodium and potassium and their intakes should not exceed 80 mmol and 50 mmol respectively per day. Despite restriction of potassium, hyperkalaemia is almost invariable and requires active measures to restore the serum potassium to normal while awaiting dialysis or between dialyses. The danger of hyperkalaemia is ventricular fibrillation, and ECG monitoring to detect early changes and measurement of serum potassium are useful. Figure 9.1 shows the typical ECG changes associated with hyperkalaemia.

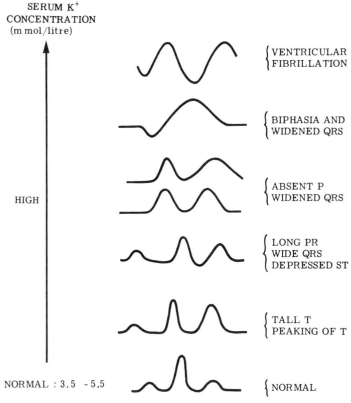

SERUM K$^+$
CONCENTRATION
(m mol/litre)

{ VENTRICULAR
FIBRILLATION

{ BIPHASIA AND
WIDENED QRS

{ ABSENT P
WIDENED QRS

HIGH

{ LONG PR
WIDE QRS
DEPRESSED ST

{ TALL T
PEAKING OF T

NORMAL : 3.5 - 5.5

{ NORMAL

FIG. 9.1 As the serum potassium rises, ECG changes develop culminating in ventricular fibrillation.

Treatment of hyperkalaemia. The measures available to treat hyperkalaemia are as follows:

1. 20 ml of 10 per cent calcium gluconate intravenously.
2. 20 units of insulin with 40 g glucose intravenously.

3. Ion exchange resin (15–30 g of calcium resonium) orally.
4. Alkali (sodium bicarbonate) intravenously.
5. Dialysis.

Intravenous calcium does not influence the serum potassium but has a protective effect on the heart and is therefore useful as an additional measure in the presence of a very high serum level. Insulin acts by promoting transfer of potassium from the extracellular fluid into the cells and is a rapid and effective measure. It is the standard emergency treatment of hyperkalaemia with a duration of action of a few hours, and is given with glucose to avoid hypoglycaemia. If required, it can be followed by the use of an ion exchange resin such as calcium resonium which is slow to act but will exert an effect over 12 hours or longer. Finally, an alkali such as sodium bicarbonate acts by correcting acidosis and therefore promoting the entry of potassium into the cells in exchange for H^+. It is not effective enough to be used alone in the treatment of hyperkalaemia.

Nutrition

There is no place for protein restriction in ARF. In the less seriously ill patient who can eat, the diet should contain about 1·25 g of protein/kg body wt/day and at least 2000 kcal/day. The ill patient who is anorexic, semi-conscious, or on a ventilator should be fed by naso-gastric tube or intravenously. For the naso-gastric feeding, one can use a solid diet which is homogenised in the ward kitchen, or commercially prepared cans of liquid food. Intravenous feeding uses amino acid preparations and calorie sources such as 50 per cent dextrose and fat emulsions. In view of the tissue breakdown in seriously ill patients, at least 2500 kilocalories and about 1·5 g protein per kg are needed daily. When amino acid preparations are used, the equivalent nitrogen content for the average sized patient is about 15 g. Such feeding regimes require a daily fluid intake of two to three litres. Blood glucose monitoring is necessary and insulin may be required to control hyperglycaemia resulting from the use of concentrated dextrose solutions.

Anaemia

A progressive fall in haemoglobin is inevitable and blood

transfusion is usually required. The aim should be to maintain the haemoglobin at around 9–10 g/100 ml.

Drug therapy

The route of elimination of any drugs used should be known. Reduction of the dose will be necessary if the drug is excreted by the kidney and if high blood levels produce toxic effects. Adjustment of the dose should also take into account any elimination of the drug by dialysis. The serum levels of some drugs can be measured, e.g. digoxin and gentamicin. Finally, nephrotoxic drugs such as tetracycline and cephaloridine should be avoided (see Table 13.1).

DIALYSIS

In view of its greater efficiency, haemodialysis is the method of choice in older children and adults although peritoneal dialysis is superior for young children. Should haemodialysis not be available, peritoneal dialysis can be used but a better option usually is the transfer of the patient to a renal unit with haemodialysis facilities. Also there are certain contraindications to peritoneal dialysis which should be observed:

1. Rapidly rising blood urea.
2. Acute or chronic respiratory failure.
3. Paralytic ileus.
4. Recent abdominal surgery.
5. Severe hypoalbuminaemia.

To obtain vessel access for haemodialysis, an arteriovenous shunt is usually inserted but a cannula in the femoral vein can be used for short periods. The need for dialysis is decided mainly on biochemical grounds as the aim is to keep the blood urea below a level which is likely to produce clinical features of uraemia. Thus the peak blood urea should be kept below 35 mmol/l and in hypercatabolic patients this usually requires daily haemodialysis. As the amount of catabolism lessens, the frequency can sometimes be reduced to alternate days. Ultrafiltration consists of the removal of water from the blood by creating a pressure gradient across the dialysis membrane. The removal of urea and other metabolites by dialysis will reduce the serum osmolality while water removal by ultrafiltration will reduce the blood volume. If these two processes are carried out together, hypotension will usually result in the ill patient with ARF. Thus most dialysis machines are now designed so that the two processes can be separated in time. With such separation, fluid can usually be removed surprisingly rapidly, up to 1500 ml per hour without causing hypotension. The removal of fluid enables adequate nutrition to be given as described above. With daily dialysis the duration of each session is usually about three hours.

COMPLICATIONS

Infection

Infection due to depression of the immune response by uraemia is a common complication. Prevention, which is aided by isolation in a single cubicle, and early diagnosis by frequent bacteriological monitoring are important aims. Antibiotic therapy should be chosen with care, bearing in mind the mode of drug metabolism. Also the impaired immune response usually demands an active surgical approach to foci of infection.

Gastrointestinal bleeding

The usual sources are gastric erosions and the mortality used to be high. Nowadays, cimetidine will control the bleeding in most cases and surgery is seldom required. The usual dose of cimetidine is 1 gram per day but half this dose will provide effective blood levels in renal failure.

Cardiac failure

This used to be a common complication due mainly to an excessive fluid intake. Good control of fluid balance and the use, when necessary, of ultrafiltration will usually avoid this problem.

Wound healing

This will be slower than normal in post-operative patients.

CAUSES OF DEATH

The initiating illness, or non-renal complications arising from it, are responsible for nearly two-thirds of deaths. The main cause of death related to the uraemic state is infection followed by a few others which should usually be preventable such as gastrointestinal bleeding, cardiac failure and hyperkalaemia.

PROGNOSIS

The overall survival rate in ATN is around 50 per cent, but this average figure conceals a wide range. In clinical practice a distinction can be made between the patient with multiple organ failure usually requiring mechanical ventilation and nursing in an intensive therapy unit, and the one whose renal failure is the main problem and who can be nursed in a conventional ward area. The recovery rate in the former group rarely exceeds 35 per cent and is often lower, while in the latter it is often around 65 per cent. Further subdivision of patients into three clinical categories gives a survival rate of about 35 per cent for the surgical group, 70 per cent for the medical group and 90 per cent for the small obstetric group. The main adverse prognostic factors are old age, uncontrolled sepsis, usually intra-abdominal, and an upper gastrointestinal lesion as the cause of the ATN.

Miscellaneous causes of ARF

These are listed on page 162 with the number of the chapter in which they are discussed. The few not covered in other chapters are considered here.

HEPATORENAL SYNDROME

This term should be reserved for the association of acute renal failure and end-stage hepatic cirrhosis. The urine findings differ from ATN in that the sodium concentration is very low (usually less than 10 mmol/l), and the urine osmolality fairly high. All that one can say about the pathogenesis is that there is a renal haemodynamic disturbance. Precipitating factors include diuretic therapy, abdominal paracentesis and gastrointestinal haemorrhage. Management consists mainly of blood volume expansion with salt-poor albumin and the avoidance of sodium administration. Dialysis is usually not indicated as the liver disease is almost always in a terminal stage. This syndrome should be distinguished from the other associations between hepatic disease and renal failure which are:

1. The combined effect of toxins on the liver and kidney, e.g. organic solvents and paracetamol overdose.
2. The increased predisposition of the kidney to ATN in jaundiced patients.
3. The occurrence of ARF in fulminant hepatic failure.
4. The involvement of liver and kidneys by multi-system disease, e.g. vasculitis.

INTRATUBULAR OBSTRUCTION

The most common cause is precipitation of uric acid following chemotherapy for haematological neoplasia. Prophylaxis consists of prior alkalinisation of the urine and use of allopurinol, and treatment, should renal failure develop, is along standard lines. Methotrexate, when used in large doses, has been reported to crystallise in the distal nephron.

SEVERE HYPERCALCAEMIA

Hypercalcaemia of sufficient severity to cause ARF is most often seen in association with a malignant tumour. Steroid therapy, e.g. prednisolone 1–2 mg/kg/day, sometimes lowers the serum calcium but only after a few days. Rapid lowering is essential to minimise renal damage and if some renal function remains, repeated doses of frusemide will produce a useful degree of elimination of calcium. Also phosphate infusions will lower the serum calcium. On theoretical grounds calcitonin should be useful but has proved disappointing in practice. In the presence of established renal failure, dialysis will lower the serum calcium as well as controlling the uraemia.

Thrombosis

ARTERIAL THROMBOSIS

Renal artery thrombosis is uncommon and the usual clinical setting is an elderly patient with widespread atheroma. The presenting features are loin pain, haematuria and, if it occurs in a solitary kidney, anuria. Thrombectomy is occasionally successful but infarction of the kidney will usually have taken place before surgery can be undertaken.

VENOUS THROMBOSIS

Renal vein thrombosis is uncommon in the adult but may follow dehydration in infancy. It may be bilateral and complete and if so will cause ARF, often with leg oedema due to associated inferior vena cava thrombosis. Renal vein thrombosis in adults is rare and usually secondary to pre-existing glomerular disease, particularly membranous nephropathy and amyloidosis. Anticoagulants are usually indicated but surgical removal of thrombus is seldom feasible.

POINTS OF EMPHASIS

● The management of pre-renal ARF should be directed at the patient's circulation and not the kidney.

● Although uncommon, it is important to exclude obstruction as a cause of ARF in patients with a suggestive presentation.

● ATN is by far the most common cause of intrinsic acute renal failure.

● ATN of ischaemic type may occur in any situation causing hypotension of sufficient duration and severity, particularly in patients predisposed by such factors as old age or sodium depletion.

● Nephrotoxic antibiotics can induce ATN at therapeutic levels and are best avoided in patients at high risk.

● Paracetamol in overdosage and paraquat are two relatively common causes of nephrotoxic ATN.

● A urine/plasma osmolality ratio of less than 1·1:1 implies ATN whereas a ratio of greater than 1·7:1 implies pre-renal failure.

● Oliguria is a common but not invariable feature of ATN.

- The clinical consequences of ARF are usually over-shadowed by the features of the illness causing the renal failure.

- During the oliguric phase, wound healing and resistance to infection are markedly depressed.

- Serious complications and death may still occur during the diuretic phase of ARF.

- Management of pre-renal ARF involves restoring the circulating blood volume. In incipient ATN, dopamine may improve renal blood flow and a trial of a diuretic such as mannitol may be of value.

- In established ATN, daily weighing is the best method of monitoring fluid balance.

- Hyperkalaemia may lead to ventricular fibrillation and is therefore highly dangerous.

- Good nutrition is essential and should consist of a high calorie, high protein diet. Intravenous feeding may be required.

- The primary indication for dialysis is biochemical; the aim is to maintain the blood urea below a level likely to produce the clinical features of uraemia.

- Haemodialysis is preferred to peritoneal dialysis except in early childhood.

- Ultrafiltration is of value in the treatment of fluid overload.

- Cimetidine is usually effective in the control of haemorrhage from gastric erosions.

- The overall mortality due to ATN is about 50 per cent but the initiating illness or associated non-renal complications are responsible for nearly two-thirds of the deaths.

CHAPTER 10

Chronic renal failure

CAUSES

There are numerous causes of chronic renal failure (CRF) but only a few common ones. Table 10.1 shows the more common causes in the young and middle-aged adult based on the data of the European Dialysis and Transplant Association. The two common diseases, glomerulonephritis in its various forms and chronic pyelonephritis, together account for just over half while the less common causes make up the remainder. One important although infrequent cause not listed separately in Table 10.1 is urinary tract obstruction which may be either mechanical or neurological and can be caused by congenital abnormalities in the young, calculi at any age and prostatic enlargement in the elderly. The miscellaneous causes include gout, hypercalcaemia, radiation and myeloma.

PATHOPHYSIOLOGY

The functions of the kidney can be divided into four groups, namely the excretion of nitrogenous waste products and acid, the control of water and electrolyte balance, the secretion of hormones and the metabolism of various compounds such as the hydroxylation of Vitamin D. The disturbances seen in CRF will be discussed under these headings.

Azotaemia and acidosis

As nephrons become damaged and cease to function, the

TABLE 10.1   Common causes of chronic renal failure.

Disease group	Incidence (per cent)
Glomerulonephritis	33
Pyelonephritis	21
Cystic disease (mainly adult polycystic kidneys)	9
Multisystem disease (mainly diabetes mellitus, also SLE and amyloid)	8
Vascular disease (mainly malignant hypertension)	8
Drug toxicity (mainly phenacetin)	3
Hereditary (e.g. hereditary nephritis)	3
Miscellaneous	15
Total	100

glomerular filtration rate (GFR) will fall and once it is below 50 per cent of normal, the serum concentration of nitrogenous end products will rise. This acts as a compensatory phenomenon to increase the filtered load of these substances and restore equilibrium. Urea is quantitatively the most important end product, while others include creatinine, uric acid and phosphate. In addition to these, which are easily measured, there are many others of larger molecular size which cannot be measured but which are probably at least as toxic as urea, and may be more so, and to which the name 'middle molecules' has been applied. The toxic effect of all these end products is widespread, involving the gastrointestinal tract with nausea and vomiting, the nervous system with neuropathy and convulsions, the pericardium with pericarditis and the skin with pruritus.

The metabolic acidosis of uraemia is contributed to in varying degree by impairment of all three renal mechanisms for maintenance of acid–base balance. The most important defect is a decrease in the excretion of the ammonium ion due to loss of healthy tubular cells needed for ammonia synthesis. The filtered load of phosphate falls, leading to reduced availability of buffer, and reabsorption of bicarbonate by the tubules becomes less complete.

The end result is metabolic acidosis with low blood pH, bicarbonate and P_{CO_2}.

Water and electrolyte balance

There is an increased solute load to each remaining healthy nephron due to the elevated blood level of nitrogenous end products. The osmotic effect of this reduces electrolyte and water reabsorption so that an osmotic diuresis with polyuria is a common feature of CRF. The maintenance of a normal or increased urine flow despite a reduction in the number of nephrons indicates an increased flow through each nephron and this reduces time-limited reabsorption. As a consequence there is impaired efficiency of the countercurrent multiplier system because of reduced medullary hypertonicity. Thus urine concentrating and diluting power are both reduced. In addition, where the renal damage affects the tubules to a greater degree than the glomeruli such as in chronic pyelonephritis, sodium and/or potassium reabsorption may be markedly impaired leading to sodium or potassium depletion and the need for dietary supplements. Urine electrolyte studies may therefore help to define the main site of renal damage.

Hormones

HORMONES SECRETED BY THE KIDNEY

Erythropoietin

While accurate techniques for measurement of erythropoietin are not yet available, there is some evidence that blood levels tend to be low in CRF. However, it is far from certain that the disturbance of erythropoietin is a simple deficiency.

Renin

This enzyme is produced by the juxtaglomerular apparatus and acts on the substrate angiotensinogen to produce angiotensin I which in turn is acted on by converting enzyme to produce angiotensin II. Renin levels may be normal or elevated in CRF and this is discussed further in the section dealing with hypertension.

HORMONES SECRETED ELSEWHERE

Abnormalities have been described in a wide variety of hormones in CRF. The serum levels of parathyroid hormone, gastrin, prolactin, glucagon and growth hormone are usually elevated while those of insulin and aldosterone may be normal or high. Thyroxine levels are usually low; of the hormones related to sexual function, testosterone and oestrogens tend to be low while luteinising hormone is usually high.

Miscellaneous metabolic functions

One of the most important of these relates to Vitamin D and this will be discussed on page 187.

CLINICAL FEATURES

Symptoms

The most common presenting symptoms of CRF are tiredness and malaise. Gastrointestinal symptoms often come next, namely anorexia, nausea and vomiting with resultant weight loss but diarrhoea is usually a late feature. Symptoms of cardiac failure include dyspnoea and ankle swelling. A distressing itch is also common. Peripheral neuropathy may occur in long-standing uraemia often presenting with the 'restless leg syndrome', an ill-defined sensation of discomfort partially relieved by movement. This may be followed by parasthesiae and later weakness. Symptoms which are less often volunteered relate to the urinary tract and sexual function. The former includes nocturia and polyuria and may lead to water depletion with thirst. The latter includes amenorrhoea in the female, impotence in the male, and loss of libido in both sexes.

Enquiry into the past history should include any routine medical examinations such as noting the presence of hypertension and/or proteinuria—these would suggest previous occult renal disease. A thorough enquiry into excessive drug use is important although the most common offender, phenacetin, has now been withdrawn from sale and therefore this cause of renal failure is becoming less common. The family history may give a lead as in polycystic kidneys and hereditary nephritis and occasionally there is a relevant occupational history such as exposure to heavy metals such as cadmium, which is nephrotoxic, or hydrocarbons, which have been implicated in some cases of glomerulonephritis.

Examination

The most common feature on general examination is pallor which may be accompanied by a yellow pigmentation, excoriation and bruising. Hypertension is very common and careful fundoscopy examination is important. Cardiac failure and cardiomegaly are also common findings and in advanced uraemia, pericardial friction is frequently heard. The peripheral neuropathy of long-standing CRF is usually initially sensory, while drowsiness, convulsions and finally coma indicate very advanced uraemia. Severe acidosis is accompanied by deep, sighing respiration known as Kussmaul breathing. The kidneys themselves are usually small or normal in size and therefore impalpable unless the patient is very thin. The notable exception is polycystic disease where the kidneys are enlarged, sometimes grossly so, one often more than the other, and with an irregular and knobbly character. Finally, the examination of a middle-aged or elderly male must include a rectal examination to assess prostatic size as prostatic obstruction is not always accompanied by the classical symptoms such as dribbling and hesitancy of micturition.

ASSESSMENT

This has four main aims, the differentiation of chronic from acute renal failure, definition of the aetiology, recognition of any potentially remediable factors and determination of the severity of the renal failure.

Differentiation from ARF

Table 10.2 lists on the left the features which are pathognomonic of CRF and also those which are suggestive but not conclusive findings. Features suggestive of ARF are shown on the right but this condition does not possess any pathognomonic findings. The differentiation of acute from chronic renal failure is also discussed in Chapter 9.

TABLE 10.2   Differentiation of acute and chronic renal failure.

	CRF	ARF
Pathognomonic features	Small kidneys on IVU Presence of chronic renal failure in the past Complications, e.g. osteodystrophy or neuropathy	None
Suggestive features	Hypertension Severe anaemia Long history of such symptoms as nocturia, thirst, pruritus, anorexia and nausea	Preceding acute incident, e.g. shock Oliguria Anaemia, mild or absent

Aetiology

In the case of the less common causes of CRF, a strong lead can usually be obtained from the history and examination. Examples are the family history in polycystic kidneys and hereditary nephritis, the drug history in analgesic nephropathy and also clear leads in diabetes mellitus, SLE and amyloid. Repeated questioning of the patient and relatives is sometimes required before the abuse of drugs such as analgesics will be admitted. Physical examination is useful in the diagnosis of polycystic kidneys, malignant hypertension and SLE. The most difficult differentiation on clinical grounds is between the two most common causes of CRF, glomerulonephritis and pyelonephritis. The absence of hypertension makes the former unlikely but, if present, is of no diagnostic help. Investigation is usually required to differentiate between these two conditions as well as to confirm other diagnoses which have been suggested by clinical features. The most useful investigations are as follows:

URINE PROTEIN

Diseases affecting mainly the glomeruli (e.g. glomerulonephritis, diabetes and amyloid) usually cause proteinuria of more than 3 grams per day, while predominantly tubular diseases (e.g. pyelonephritis, polycystic kidneys and analgesic nephropathy) are associated with less than 1·5 grams per day.

SERUM BIOCHEMISTRY

For a comparable degree of uraemia, predominantly tubular diseases give rise to a more severe degree of acidosis (Table 10.3). Also, but less consistently, tubular diseases tend to be associated with sodium and/or potassium depletion which may be reflected in the serum biochemistry.

TABLE 10.3   Typical serum biochemistry values in chronic renal failure.

Serum biochemistry values (mmol/l)	Glomerular disease (e.g. glomerulonephritis)	Tubular disease (e.g. chronic pyelonephritis)
Na^+	140	130
K^+	4·8	3·6
Cl^-	96	102
HCO_3^-	20	12
Urea	40	38

INTRAVENOUS UROGRAPHY (IVU)

A high dose of contrast and the use of tomography will often yield valuable information as discussed in Chapter 2. Table 10.4 shows the most frequent abnormalities seen.

OTHER RADIOLOGICAL STUDIES

A retrograde pyelogram may be of value in hydronephrosis, ureteric obstruction, papillary necrosis or polycystic kidneys, but is often unnecessary if the IVU is of good quality. An arteriogram will confirm renal artery stenosis.

ULTRASOUND

This is most useful in obstructive conditions and polycystic kidneys,

TABLE 10.4 IVU in chronic renal failure.

Abnormality	Diagnosis
Symmetrical reduction in renal size	Glomerulonephritis Malignant hypertension
Asymmetrical reduction in renal size — Normal calyces — Clubbed calyces with cortical scars	Unilateral ischaemia, e.g. renal artery stenosis Pyelonephritis
Papillary necrosis	Analgesic nephropathy
Very large kidneys with irregular outline	Polycystic kidneys
Generalised calyceal dilatation	Obstructive lesion
Normal renal size and calyces	Amyloid or other glomerular lesion of fairly recent onset

and in both of these is of greater diagnostic value than an IVU if renal function is very poor.

RENAL BIOPSY

The usual indication for a biopsy in renal failure is the presence of normal or slightly reduced kidneys where all other tests have failed to establish a diagnosis. A kidney which is considerably reduced in size (e.g. less than 11 cm in length in an adult of average size) should not usually be biopsied by the percutaneous method as there is an increased risk of bleeding. Biopsy is of much less value in CRF than in renal failure of recent onset as the histological appearances are often non-specific.

Remediable factors

The only cause of CRF which is to a considerable extent remediable is urinary tract obstruction. In addition, there are a number of factors which can add to the severity of renal failure and which are to a variable degree reversible.

FLUID AND/OR ELECTROLYTE DEPLETION

The depletion most commonly found is of sodium and potassium. The site of loss is either the kidney, due to tubular damage with a resultant 'leak', or the gastrointestinal tract, due to vomiting and/or diarrhoea.

INFECTION

Deterioration in renal function can occur either in infection within the urinary tract, if this ascends to the kidneys, or in infection elsewhere.

CARDIAC FAILURE

While this is a frequent complication it is seldom possible to improve cardiac function to any great extent.

DRUGS

The most frequent offenders are antibiotics such as cephalosporins, aminoglycosides and cotrimoxazole. All drugs should be prescribed with great care to patients with CRF (see Table 13.1).

BLOOD PRESSURE

While a poorly controlled blood pressure and particularly malignant hypertension will accelerate deterioration in renal function, an improvement in control will seldom result in any major recovery of renal function. Exceptions to this general rule occur and occasionally considerable improvement in renal function is seen following control of malignant hypertension.

Severity of renal failure

This is determined by measurement of glomerular filtration rate (GFR). The blood urea and serum creatinine provide an indirect measurement while the creatinine clearance gives a more direct measurement. It should be appreciated that the blood urea is influenced by the rate of urea production and therefore by both dietary protein intake and the rate of endogenous protein breakdown. Thus while it may not accurately reflect GFR it is still useful as an index of the severity of uraemia and therefore the need for treatment. Serum creatinine measurement correlates well with GFR and is a better guide than blood urea although it may be falsely low in patients who have lost a considerable amount of lean body mass, and it may also be transiently elevated following the ingestion of cooked meat. Finally, while the creatinine clearance does not correlate perfectly with GFR, it is accurate enough for routine clinical practice.

COURSE

Although one can only give general guidance, some prediction can be made of the likely rate of progression with the different causes of CRF. At one end of the spectrum is polycystic kidney disease in which renal function may deteriorate over two decades or more. In chronic pyelonephritis, also, advanced renal failure may be reached

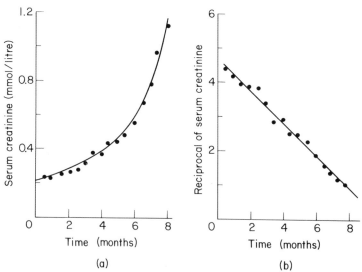

(a)   (b)

FIG. 10.1   (a) Serial serum creatinine measurements in a patient with progressive chronic renal failure.
(b) Plotting the reciprocal of the serum creatinine gives a straight line which allows more accurate prediction of the time when end-stage renal failure will be reached.

after ten or more years. At the other end of the spectrum CRF merges with ARF, for example in malignant hypertension and rapidly progressive glomerulonephritis. In between are most cases of glomerulonephritis, diabetic nephropathy and amyloid where advanced renal failure is reached a few years from the time renal function first becomes impaired.

The rate of progression is best measured by serial serum creatinine or creatinine clearance estimations. When plotted against time, the values for serum creatinine usually lie along a curve (Figure 10.1a). If the reciprocal is plotted instead, a straight line is obtained (Fig. 10.1b) which allows more accurate prediction of when the patient will reach end-stage renal failure.

COMPLICATIONS

Osteodystrophy

PATHOPHYSIOLOGY

The term osteodystrophy includes all types of bone disease seen in CRF. Before discussing these individually, their pathophysiology will be reviewed, in which there are two important initiating events. The first relates to vitamin D metabolism. Cholecalciferol is obtained in the diet and formed from the effect of sunlight on the skin. It is hydroxylated in the liver to 25-hydroxycholecalciferol (25-HCC). This is further hydroxylated in the kidney to 1,25-dihydroxycholecalciferol (1,25-DHCC), which is the main active metabolite. With increasing renal damage the kidney produces less 1,25-DHCC resulting in a reduction of calcium absorption and therefore hypocalcaemia. The second event is the reduction of phosphorus excretion which begins when the GFR falls to around half of normal and which tends to raise the serum phosphorus. Both the hypocalcaemia and the tendency for the serum phosphorus to rise stimulate the parathyroid glands and this begins at a fairly early stage of the renal failure. The serum parathyroid hormone (PTH) level can now be accurately measured by radioimmunoassay and as renal failure reaches an advanced stage, high serum PTH levels can be demonstrated, confirming the presence of secondary hyperparathyroidism (Fig. 10.2). There are three important end results of these sequences of events.

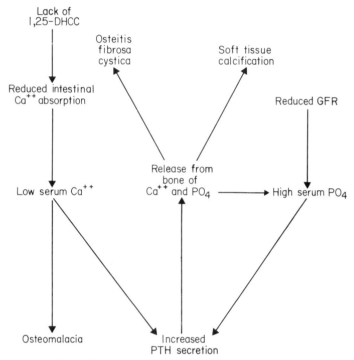

FIG. 10.2   Pathogenesis of renal osteodystrophy.

SECONDARY HYPERPARATHYROIDISM (OSTEITIS FIBROSA CYSTICA)

The bone changes are usually asymptomatic and consist of subperiosteal erosions seen best on X-ray of the phalanges (Fig. 10.3). Later a 'ground glass' appearance may be seen in the skull and larger cystic areas develop in other bones. The serum alkaline phosphatase is usually elevated.

OSTEOMALACIA

In most patients, the radiological and histological changes of this (or rickets in the child) coexist with those of hyperparathyroidism and can be attributed to the deficiency of 1,25-DHCC and resultant hypocalcaemia. Unlike hyperparathyroidism, osteomalacia may

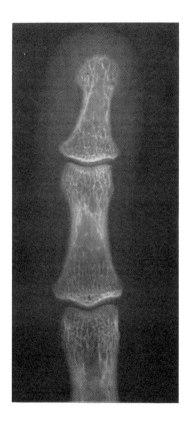

FIG. 10.3 A magnified radiograph of a phalanx in secondary hyperparathyroidism showing the subperiosteal resorption of bone, most marked in the middle phalanx and at the tip of the terminal phalanx.

cause bone pain and deformity and a myopathy with muscle weakness.

SOFT TISSUE CALCIFICATION

This will occur if the serum calcium and phosphorus product (expressed in mmol/l) is consistently greater than 5·5. As the phosphorus level is elevated in CRF much more than the calcium is depressed, this complication results from a consistently high serum phosphorus. There are four common sites of deposition. Periarticular calcification most often occurs around the shoulders and in the hands. It may cause acute pain similar to gout and has thus been termed pseudogout. Conjunctival calcification can cause inflammation leading to the condition of 'red eye'. In the cornea, the deposition is asymptomatic but can be seen as band keratopathy. Finally vascular calcification initially involves the distal arteries of the limbs and later more proximal arteries. This can lead to serious difficulties in creating vessel access for dialysis and carrying out the vascular surgery required during transplantation.

Two other bone abnormalities are seen in CRF which cannot be directly attributed to the events outlined in Figure 10.2.

OSTEOSCLEROSIS

This is diagnosed radiologically, consists of areas of increased bone density, and is of unknown cause although fairly common. It is recognised most often in the lumbar spine where horizontal sclerotic bands alternate with bands of normal or reduced bone density giving rise to the appearance named 'rugger jersey spine'.

OSTEOPOROSIS

It is difficult both to define the aetiology and to diagnose osteoporosis. It may lead to backache and pathological fractures, and can be suspected from decreased bone density on X-ray. Confirmation can be provided by isotope studies which measure the calcium content of bone.

TREATMENT

The first step in the treatment of osteodystrophy is to lower the serum phosphorus by binding dietary phosphorus with aluminium hydroxide thus preventing its absorption. Aludrox gel or tablets or Alucap capsules can be used and should be taken about 15 minutes before meals in a dose of 3–15 tablets (15–75 ml Aludrox gel) per day. Evidence is accumulating that some absorbtion of aluminium occurs from the intestine and other phosphate binding agents are being evaluated. A serum phosphorus of 2 mmol/l is often taken as the concentration above which aluminium hydroxide is indicated, with the aim of maintaining it below this level. Once this has been achieved, it is safe to prescribe Vitamin D either in the form of 1 α-cholecalciferol which is converted in the liver to 1,25-DHCC or by giving 1,25-DHCC itself. Both these compounds are effective but they can produce deterioration of renal function even in the absence of hypercalcaemia. They should, therefore, only be used in the patient not yet on dialysis if there is biochemical or radiological evidence of severe hyperparathyroidism and the maintenance dose should be as low as possible, usually 0·25–0·5 μg per day. Once on long term dialysis, there is virtually no renal function to conserve and these vitamin D analogues should then be used even with mild hyperparathyroidism although still with frequent monitoring to avoid hypercalcaemia. While hyperparathyroidism usually responds well as judged by radiological or biochemical criteria, histological improvement is less consistent. Also severe hyperparathyroidism may not respond at all and require subtotal parathyroidectomy. This operation consists usually of removal of three glands and half of the fourth and is indicated in the presence of persisting hyperparathyroidism with a very high serum PTH level which has not been suppressed by 1 α-cholecalciferol or when this compound leads to hypercalcaemia despite failure to suppress the parathyroid glands. The hyperparathyroidism may also lead to failure of control of the serum phosphorus despite aluminium hydroxide. Osteomalacia responds much less well than hyperparathyroidism to 1 α-cholecalciferol and probably osteoporosis and osteosclerosis do not benefit at all.

Anaemia

This usually develops once the GFR has fallen below half normal and becomes more severe as renal function deteriorates. A few patients, particularly those with polycystic kidneys, are able to maintain a near normal haemoglobin despite advanced renal failure. Reduced erythropoietin secretion and possibly also circulating antagonists to erythropoietin result in impaired red cell production by the marrow. In addition, the red cells which are formed have a reduced life span. Iron stores are usually normal except in haemodialysis patients in whom blood loss related to the dialysis procedure may result in iron deficiency. The typical blood film is normochromic but shows anisocytosis and poikilocytosis and sometimes crenated cells known as burr cells. Anaemia plays a major role in the ill health of the renal failure patient contributing to the tiredness, exertional dyspnoea and cardiac failure. Management consists of the administration of oral iron and folic acid if the diet is restricted or the patient on haemodialysis. Blood transfusion is given for severe, symptomatic anaemia and is not usually required until the haemoglobin has fallen below 7 g/100 ml. If possible frozen, thawed red cells should be used to minimise the risk of hepatitis transmission and reduce the incidence of sensitisation to HLA antigens when repeated transfusion is required. There is a risk of haemosiderosis with repeated transfusions but the number of units required by most patients makes this risk more theoretical than real.

Neurological complications

Two complications which may affect the nervous system are neuropathy and encephalopathy.

NEUROPATHY

Almost all patients with moderate or advanced renal failure will have prolonged motor nerve conduction velocities on testing but only a minority have clinical abnormalities and very few have severe neuropathy. The 'restless leg syndrome' is often the first manifestation of sensory disturbance and consists of unpleasant pruritic and prickling sensations occurring mainly in the lower limbs at night. Other abnormal sensations such as burning feet also occur with motor neuropathy only in more advanced cases. Neuropathy does not respond to any dietary or drug regime. It may be slightly improved or at least arrested by long-term haemodialysis and will usually resolve after successful transplantation.

ENCEPHALOPATHY

Obvious abnormalities only occur in advanced uraemia although careful testing will show changes at an earlier stage. These early changes include impaired concentrating power, mild confusion and loss of memory, leading eventually to delirium. Other features which may occur are a flapping tremor, muscle twitching (myoclonus) and tetany. Generalised motor or sometimes focal convulsions may occur at a late stage. The causes are probably multiple including accumulation of uraemic toxins. Convulsions may also be precipitated by the lowering of serum ionised calcium which can follow the rapid correction of acidosis with sodium bicarbonate and this measure is not advisable in the presence of a very low serum calcium. Convulsions are treated with anticonvulsants and calcium infusions in the circumstances just described.

Hypertension

This complication is frequent and its incidence is related to the cause of the renal failure. For example almost all patients with advanced renal failure due to glomerulonephritis are hypertensive but many with chronic pyelonephritis are not.

The mechanism of blood pressure control in the normal person is highly complex but it is clear that there are two factors of particular importance, the body sodium content and the renin–angiotensin system. Plasma renin correlates closely with angiotensin II and they both show an inverse relation with total body sodium (Fig. 10.4) in normotensive subjects with or without renal failure. In most patients with hypertension and renal failure, total body sodium is raised and also the plasma renin is usually high in relation to body sodium but falls to normal with effective treatment. Persistence of high plasma renin levels often correlates with resistance to treatment.

Hypertension has an important influence on the course of CRF. Renal function will usually deteriorate rapidly in the presence of poor blood pressure control and especially malignant phase hypertension. Also the malignant phase is relatively more common when the hypertension is of renal origin than in essential hypertension. As renal function deteriorates, blood pressure

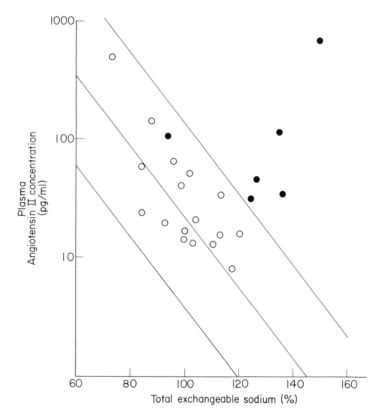

FIG. 10.4   In normotensive patients with or without renal failure (○)
there is an inverse relationship between plasma angiotensin II and total
exchangeable body sodium. In patients with hypertension and
renal failure (●) the plasma angiotensin II is high in relation to body
sodium.

tends to rise further and a vicious circle may become established.

The hypertension of CRF is commonly resistant to treatment and
the drugs listed in Table 10.5 frequently have to be used in
combination. A beta blocker is usually the first choice provided
there is no evidence of cardiac failure. Its action in lowering cardiac
output will tend to reduce renal blood flow and there have been
reports of deterioration in renal function in renal failure patients
receiving beta blockers. By contrast nadolol, a newer non-selective
beta blocker, has been shown to increase renal blood flow and if

TABLE 10.5 Antihypertensive therapy in chronic renal failure.

Name	Mode of action	Dose range (mg day)
First line drugs		
Propranolol	Non-selective beta blocker	20–2000
Oxprenolol	Non-selective beta blocker	40–2000
Nadolol	Non-selective beta blocker	40–640
Metoprolol	Selective beta blocker	200–600
Atenolol	Selective beta blocker	100–400
Labetalol	Alpha and beta blocker	300–2400
Hydralazine.	Vasodilator	50–200
Second line drugs		
Prazosin	Vasodilator	1·5–20
Clonidine	Central action and alpha blocker	0·1–1·2
Drugs for resistant hypertension		
Minoxidil	Vasodilator	5–60
Captopril	Angiotensin converting enzyme inhibitor	25–450

further studies confirm this, it will have a useful role in renal failure. The combination of alpha and beta blockade also gives labetalol an advantage over the remaining beta blockers. In mild renal failure, the addition of a thiazide or xipamide is useful while in advanced CRF frusemide is preferable due to its greater diuretic potency although its intrinsic antihypertensive effect may be less than that of a thiazide. The use of a vasodilator such as hydralazine or prazosin in addition to a beta blocker and diuretic is the next step if blood pressure control remains poor. Clonidine, which acts centrally, can also be given but is usually less effective. Minoxidil, which is a potent vasodilator, can be substituted in resistant cases for the vasodilator already in use. It is highly effective but has two disadvantages, hirsutism which may be unacceptable in females, and sodium retention which can usually be controlled by high dose frusemide. Finally, converting enzyme antagonists, which reduce the production of angiotension II, are now available, the first of which is captopril. They offer hope of improved blood pressure control in patients with resistant hypertension due to excess renin production.

Cardiovascular complications

These are very important numerically, accounting for much ill-health and about half of all deaths in chronic renal failure. They can be subdivided into four groups.

VASCULAR DISEASE

The frequent occurrence of two important risk factors, hyperlipidaemia and hypertension, undoubtedly play a part in the high incidence of vascular disease in CRF. The manifestations are the common ones of myocardial ischaemia, cerebrovascular accidents and peripheral vascular disease.

CARDIAC FAILURE

This also is very common in CRF with several contributory factors. These include hypertension, anaemia, myocardial ischaemia and fluid and sodium retention. Left ventricular failure (LVF) is more common than right sided heart failure, evidence of the important aetiological role of hypertension and therefore one of the most important therapeutic aims must be good blood pressure control. LVF is also a fairly common initial mode of presentation in CRF. Sodium retention requires the use of a potent diuretic, frusemide being the most effective, and a dose of up to 1·5 grams per day may be needed. Because of the resistance to diuretics, a low sodium diet is also advised. Digoxin is of limited value unless in the presence of rapid atrial fibrillation. If required, the maintenance dose should be low, usually 0·0625 to 0·125 mg per day, with estimation at intervals of the serum level to avoid toxicity. Digitaxin (0·1 mg per day) is an alternative to digoxin which has the advantage of being predominantly metabolised by the liver.

PERICARDITIS

This is probably due mainly to an irritant effect of uraemic toxins on the pericardium and is commonly seen only in advanced uraemia. It is not often associated with pain but usually presents with a friction rub and sometimes later an effusion. The detection of a rub is an indication for immediate dialysis, after which it usually disappears within a few days. Ultrasound examination is the most useful technique for detecting fluid in the pericardial sac although it cannot distinguish between a serous effusion and blood. Haemorrhagic pericarditis may be precipitated by heparinisation for haemodialysis and once pericarditis has developed, heparin dosage during haemodialysis must be carefully monitored. Haemorrhagic pericarditis is extremely dangerous as it can lead to cardiac tamponade. The clinical signs of tamponade are those of circulatory failure with jugular venous congestion and sometimes pulsus paradoxus and this diagnosis should be considered in any patient with a previous friction rub who becomes acutely ill with signs of cardiac failure. Tamponade is an acute emergency which should be treated by immediate aspiration and drainage of the pericardial sac. Recurrent tamponade is an indication for pericardectomy.

ARRHYTHMIAS

The most important of these is ventricular fibrillation due to hyperkalaemia. This should be prevented by careful monitoring of the serum potassium. The management of hyperkalaemia is discussed in Chapter 8.

Infection

The immune response is of two types, cell-mediated and humoral. In uraemic patients there is clear evidence of depression of the cell-mediated response but less clear evidence regarding the humoral response, i.e. antibody production. This depression of immune response in uraemia is the major factor in the predisposition to infection. The commonest sites are the chest and urinary tract and a variety of bacteria are the usual pathogens. In addition, the depression of immune response predisposes to opportunistic infections mainly in the lungs and central nervous system and due most often to tubercle bacilli and fungi. This predisposition is shared with patients who are immunosuppressed following transplantation, and these infections are discussed under this heading in Chapter 12. The important points in management are early diagnosis with the help of the bacteriology, mycology and virology laboratories and the careful use of antibiotics and other drugs. The two main principles of drug therapy are to know how the drug is eliminated from the body and whether high serum levels are toxic. Two common examples of the use of antibiotics will be given and the subject of drug therapy is discussed in detail in Chapter 13. The penicillins are an example of a group of drugs which are excreted by the kidney and will therefore accumulate in renal failure. However, high serum levels of the penicillins are relatively non-toxic and therefore normal doses are safe although some reduction in dosage is recommended. By contrast, the aminoglycosides are ototoxic and must be given in reduced dose with daily measurement of peak and trough serum levels.

Gastrointestinal complications

Anorexia, nausea and vomiting are frequently presenting symptoms in CRF. Later features are hiccup, uraemic halitosis and diarrhoea. All these will tend to improve with institution of a low protein diet. Finally there is an increased incidence of peptic ulceration in CRF which may cause gastrointestinal bleeding.

Cutaneous features

Pallor is almost invariable in severe CRF due to the anaemia and in addition there is often yellow colouration of the skin due to the deposition of urochrome pigment. The skin may be dry and covered with scratch marks or abrasions which are self-induced because of persistent pruritus. The dryness of the skin and the patient's poor resistance to infection may combine to make boils a frequent occurrence.

Hyperlipidaemia

The increased incidence of vascular disease in CRF is due in part to the presence of hyperlipidaemia. This consists mainly of high plasma triglyceride levels largely as the very low density lipoprotein (VLDL) fraction. The pathogenesis of the hyperlipidaemia is not certain but two factors are the high carbohydrate diet which these patients often have to take to maintain energy requirements and a reduced amount of lipoprotein lipase. In theory, the serum triglyceride could be lowered by carbohydrate restriction but this is unwise in addition to restriction of dietary protein.

MANAGEMENT

This can be divided into four parts:

1. Correction of remediable factors.
2. Standard conservative measures.
3. Treatment of complications.
4. Dialysis.

The correction of remediable factors and treatment of complications have been discussed earlier in this chapter.

Standard conservative measures

These are summarised in Table 10.6.

TABLE 10.6   Conservative treatment of chronic renal failure.

Diet	Low protein (40 g), high calorie
Electrolyte intake	Variable: low Na^+ if hypertension present
Fluid intake	Usually high
Acidosis	Sodium bicarbonate
Drug therapy	Minimise use, reduce dose if necessary
Psychological state	Explanation of prognosis and treatment, and psychological support

DIET

The basic aim is to reduce the formation of nitrogenous end products by reducing protein intake but not below the minimum required to maintain positive nitrogen balance. This minimum would be 15–20 grams of protein of animal origin, in view of its high nutritional value. If of mixed animal and vegetable origin the minimum would be 30 grams. A useful standard diet in CRF contains 40 grams of protein of mixed origin as this sufficiently exceeds the minimum to avoid the risk of malnutrition. In addition, there is a limited place for a very low protein diet in patients in whom haemodialysis is not contemplated. Giordano and Giovanetti evolved such a diet which consists of 15 grams of animal protein (mainly egg) and about 3 grams of low protein foods such as vegetables or pasta to provide the bulk. This very low protein diet (the Giovanetti diet) will just maintain positive nitrogen balance as it is almost all of animal origin but is unpalatable and poorly tolerated by many patients. If adhered to it can, however, considerably lower the blood urea, with some relief from such symptoms as anorexia, nausea, vomiting and tiredness.

ELECTROLYTE INTAKE

In most patients who have a normal blood pressure, no restrictions are required until the renal failure is advanced. A few patients with predominantly tubular damage such as occurs in chronic pyelonephritis cannot conserve sodium and/or potassium and require supplements. Hypertensive patients should usually have sodium restriction.

FLUID INTAKE

As the solute concentration of the urine is fairly fixed in CRF, an increase in urine flow will increase total solute excretion. Thus a high fluid intake should usually be encouraged and this simple measure can sometimes substantially lower the blood urea.

ACIDOSIS

A reasonable general guide would be that acidosis should be corrected once the serum bicarbonate concentration has fallen to 14 mmol/l or below. Treatment usually consists of oral sodium bicarbonate in doses up to 5 grams per day. The usual tablet strength is 600 mg and an average dose is four tablets per day. Care is required if there is any tendency to sodium retention, as in cardiac failure and high doses of frusemide may be necessary. A balance may need to be struck between complete correction of acidosis and the precipitation of cardiac failure. Fortunately acidosis of a severity requiring treatment usually occurs in diseases where tubular damage predominates, such as chronic pyelonephritis, and in these cases the tendency is towards depletion of sodium rather than its retention. Rapid correction of acidosis should be avoided in patients with hypocalcaemia because of the increased liability to convulsions.

DRUG THERAPY

There are a few simple rules. Only drugs which are essential should be used. If eliminated mainly or entirely by the kidney, the dose should be reduced and if it is potentially a toxic drug, blood levels should be measured if possible. Finally there is increased potential for drug interactions so the use of multiple drugs should be kept to a minimum. This subject is discussed further in Chapter 13.

PSYCHOLOGICAL STATE

The progressive nature of the illness and the patient's realisation of the prognosis and possible eventual need for dialysis will usually induce anxiety and/or depression. Reassurance, explanation of the prognosis and treatment and psychological support are important but often neglected aspects of treatment.

Dialysis

The use of dialysis for long-term treatment of end-stage CRF is discussed in Chapter 11 and its use in ARF in Chapter 8. This leaves two aspects to be dealt with here, the use of dialysis in the initial treatment of advanced uraemia, and the treatment of 'acute on chronic' renal failure.

INITIAL TREATMENT OF ADVANCED URAEMIA

Not infrequently, the patient with CRF fails to seek medical attention until severely uraemic. In such cases, dialysis is required before detailed assessment can take place. Often left ventricular failure is present as well, precipitated by such factors as hypertension, anaemia and water and sodium overload. In most of these patients, peritoneal dialysis is the better option. Its main advantages are the simplicity of the technique and the scope for considerable fluid removal. These patients may have a fluid excess of 10–20 litres or more and this volume can be removed steadily over 24–72 hours. The uraemia will also be smoothly corrected over this time scale. Where contraindications to peritoneal dialysis exist (see list on page 171), haemodialysis can be used.

'ACUTE ON CHRONIC' RENAL FAILURE

This problem may arise in a number of ways but there are two broad categories. The first is the sudden deterioration in previously stable renal disease, e.g. due to loss of blood pressure control in hypertensive nephrosclerosis, a flare up of renal infection in chronic pyelonephritis or bleeding into polycystic kidneys. The second category is acute tubular necrosis of toxic (e.g. drug) or ischaemic origin occurring in a patient with chronic renal disease. This type of renal failure will usually improve over a few days or a few weeks provided the underlying damage is not too far advanced. The same guidance as to the best type of dialysis applies here as in acute renal failure (Chapter 8). In summary, the seriously ill patient with rapidly rising blood urea or who is likely to be oliguric for more than a week is best treated by haemodialysis. Peritoneal dialysis is satisfactory for short periods or in the less seriously ill patient.

POINTS OF EMPHASIS

- Glomerulonephritis and chronic pyelonephritis together account for just over half of all cases of CRF.

- Polyuria is a common feature of CRF.

- The most common presenting symptoms of CRF are tiredness and malaise.

- Hypertension is very common in CRF.

- The possibility of prostatic obstruction must always be considered in the middle-aged or elderly male with CRF.

- The assessment of a patient with CRF comprises differentiation from ARF, the definition of the aetiology, the recognition of any potentially remediable factor and determination of the severity of the renal failure.

● An IVU using a high dose of contrast with tomography will often yield valuable information regarding the cause of CRF.

● Potentially remediable factors are obstruction, fluid and electrolyte depletion, infection, the use of nephrotoxic drugs, cardiac failure and poorly controlled hypertension.

● The rate of progression of CRF is best measured by serial estimations of the serum creatinine or creatinine clearance.

● Osteodystrophy is due to a combination of impaired renal production of 1,25-DHCC, secondary hyperparathyroidism and hyperphosphataemia, complicated by osteosclerosis and osteoporosis.

● The first step in the treatment of osteodystrophy involves a reduction of the serum phosphorus to a concentration of less than 2 mmol/l by the administration of aluminium hydroxide.

● Vitamin D can cause a deterioration in renal function and it should only be administered with extreme caution to patients not receiving dialysis.

● Severe hyperparathyroidism may require sub-total parathyroidectomy.

● Blood transfusion should only be given for severe symptomatic anaemia.

● Neuropathy may be arrested by long-term haemodialysis and usually resolves after successful transplantation.

● Hypertension of CRF is often resistant to treatment and drug combinations are commonly required.

● Contributory factors to left ventricular failure include hypertension, anaemia, myocardial ischaemia and sodium retention.

● Left ventricular failure is a fairly common mode of presentation in CRF.

● Haemorrhagic pericarditis may be precipitated by heparinisation for dialysis and can cause cardiac tamponade.

● Pericarditis is best avoided by commencing dialysis before advanced uraemia is reached.

● Infection is common as a result of depression of the immune response by renal failure.

● A standard diet in CRF comprises 40 grams of mixed animal and vegetable protein.

● A high fluid intake should be encouraged in CRF.

● Sodium bicarbonate will correct acidosis but may precipitate cardiac failure.

● Drugs must be used with care in CRF and reduction of dosage may be necessary.

● Reassurance with explanation of the prognosis and treatment, and psychological support are important but often neglected aspects of treatment.

CHAPTER 11

Dialysis in chronic renal failure

INTRODUCTION

Modern dialysis started with the development of the artificial kidney machine by Willem Kolff in Holland during the nineteen forties. Initially its use was restricted to acute renal failure but since the introduction of the arteriovenous shunt in 1960 a vast expansion has taken place. This is shown by the rise in the number of patients on haemodialysis in Europe from 160 in 1965 to 35000 in 1979.

SELECTION

The aim should be to select for dialysis all patients in whom a reasonable quality of health can be anticipated, barring unforeseen complications. In most, this decision is easy, in some it can be very difficult. The indication for dialysis is end stage chronic renal failure which has ceased to respond to conservative management. The main guide to selection is age although this must be applied flexibly. Most patients between the ages of 5 and 70 years are suitable while most outwith this range are not. Final selection depends on the absence of adverse factors such as:

Severe vascular disease: cerebral, coronary or peripheral.
Cardiac failure.
Multisystem disease (e.g. diabetes mellitus).
Advanced uraemic complications, e.g. neuropathy.
Low IQ.
Psychosis.
Positive HBs antigen.

205

These also must not be applied too rigidly. For example, diabetes *per se* is not a contraindication but diabetes with blindness and severe cardiac disease would be. Vascular and cardiac disease form the commonest group of adverse factors while diabetes is the most frequent example of multisystem disease. SLE and amyloidosis are examples of multisystem disease which often form no contraindication to dialysis. Advanced uraemic complications which are poorly reversible such as neuropathy are very unusual. Average or high intelligence is not essential and the latter can even be a disadvantage. Sound common sense is much more useful. A patient requiring institutional care or its equivalent because of mental deficiency would almost inevitably be regarded as unsuitable. Good motivation and mental stability are clear advantages but their lack cannot be regarded as a contraindication, only a disadvantage. A psychosis, however, would almost always preclude dialysis. The last adverse factor listed, a positive HBs antigen, would rule out haemodialysis within the hospital unit but home haemodialysis or peritoneal dialysis would be practicable. Finally, selection will also be influenced by the type of dialysis contemplated. For example, the older patient with extensive peripheral vascular disease might well be unsuitable for haemodialysis because of difficulty with vessel access but be suitable for peritoneal dialysis.

TIME OF STARTING DIALYSIS

The decision to start dialysis is based on both clinical and biochemical criteria. The principle is to start prior to the stage when uraemic complications such as pericarditis or frequent vomiting are likely to arise. In practice this usually means a creatinine clearance of around 5 ml/min, or serum creatinine of more than 1200 μmol/l. The majority of patients can continue to work until, or shortly before, this level of renal function is reached. Infrequently, the presence of complicating factors such as intractable hypertension, or associated ill health due to multisystem disease such as diabetes mellitus require an earlier start. Very seldom would dialysis be contemplated before the creatinine clearance had fallen below 10 ml/min. With close observation and strict limitation of dietary protein, reasonable well-being can often be maintained without dialysis down to a creatinine clearance of 2 ml/min. While such delay may be acceptable in a few patients or to circumvent a temporary shortage of dialysis facilities, it is not generally advised.

PRINCIPLES OF DIALYSIS

Dialysis involves the use of a semi-permeable membrane across which small molecules can diffuse while larger molecules cannot. In haemodialysis, the patient's blood is pumped through an extracorporeal circuit consisting of the dialyser with its membrane. In peritoneal dialysis, the peritoneum itself acts as the dialysing membrane. Low molecular weight protein metabolites such as urea and creatinine cross the dialysis membrane freely, while higher molecular weight uraemic toxins do so less readily. In haemodialysis, the dialysis fluid circulates on the opposite side of the membrane to the blood, while in peritoneal dialysis the fluid is run into the peritoneal cavity. Dialysis fluid has an electrolyte composition similar to the physiological levels present in blood with respect to sodium, chloride, calcium and magnesium, but the potassium concentration is low to correct the hyperkalaemia which is common in renal failure. Finally acetate or lactate is present as a substitute for bicarbonate to correct acidosis.

HAEMODIALYSERS

Cellulose has been the basis of most dialysis membranes up to the present, originally in the form of Cellophane and later Cuprophan. Cellulose acetate is also widely used and a number of other membranes are being introduced or undergoing evaluation. Nowadays most renal units use disposable dialysers of the flat plate type, which has multiple layers of membrane, or the hollow fibre design which consists of a bundle of hollow fibres encased in a plastic jacket. The two other designs are the non-disposable flat plate, in which the dialyser is used repeatedly with only the membrane being renewed, and the disposable coil type, again using Cellophane or Cuprophan. Differing membrane characteristics allow the operator to vary both the clearance of molecules such as urea and the rate of water transfer across the membrane. The latter, known as ultrafiltration, is also controlled by adjustment of the pressure gradient across the membrane and is an essential component of treatment.

THE KIDNEY MACHINE

This consists of a proportioning system with associated monitoring devices. The proportioning system produces the dialysis fluid by mixing water and dialysis fluid concentrate in a ratio of around 34 to 1. The fluid is then warmed and delivered to the dialyser. Monitoring devices with incorporation of fail-safe alarm systems allow the operation of the machine by those with no technical training, including the patient. In most parts of the world it is necessary to remove calcium and other trace elements from the tap water which is used to prepare the dialysis fluid. This is probably best accomplished by reverse osmosis.

VESSEL ACCESS

Of the numerous methods which have been described, the four most useful are the arteriovenous (AV) shunt, arteriovenous (AV) fistula, vascular graft and single lumen cannula. All of these should have sufficient blood flow to provide to the dialyser a blood flow of 200 to 300 ml per min.

AV shunt

This consists of two limbs of synthetic rubber (Silastic) which form a U loop and are joined together by a connector piece between dialyses. Tapered Teflon tips are inserted into artery and vein and joined to the Silastic tubing. This device has the advantage of immediate use but its usage is often limited to a few months by the development of thrombosis or infection and it is cumbersome and unsightly. It may be inserted at the ankle or forearm.

AV fistula

This is the best long-term method. It is usually created at the wrist by anastomosis of the radial artery to the cephalic vein but can be formed higher up the arm. The increased blood flow in the venous system leads to dilatation of the veins and thickening of their walls over the subsequent few weeks. Thereafter these veins can be cannulated at two separate points to provide the blood flow to and from the dialyser.

Vascular graft

At the present time, three types are in common use. The most satisfactory material is autogenous long saphenous vein although this cannot be cannulated for several weeks until the vein wall thickens. Other options are human umbilical vein or the synthetic material Goretex. The graft can either be inserted as a U loop in the forearm or as a straight segment in the forearm or upper arm.

Cannula

As a temporary measure, a single lumen cannula can be inserted in the femoral vein and dialysis performed using a modified blood pump. The cannula is kept patent by a heparin infusion between dialyses.

Vessel access planning

If possible, an AV fistula should be created several weeks before dialysis is required. This will enable a smooth start to be made and the fistula will usually last for several years. For immediate use an AV shunt is inserted in the leg so that the vessels of the wrist can be used for creating a fistula. The vascular graft is reserved for patients in whom satisfactory AV fistulae cannot be created, while the single lumen cannula is useful for short periods of vascular access of up to a few weeks.

METHODS OF DIALYSIS

There are three main options, haemodialysis in a hospital unit, haemodialysis in the patient's home, and peritoneal dialysis.

Hospital haemodialysis

The most commonly used plan is thrice weekly dialysis, each session lasting for four to six hours. This is a compromise which allows the patient a reasonable amount of time off dialysis together with adequate although not good biochemical control. A fairly liberal protein intake can be allowed, around 1·25 g/kg body weight per day. The most important restrictions required are of sodium and potassium intake which should each be limited to 100 mmol per day or less and total fluids should not exceed about 750 ml per day with an additional allowance for any residual urine volume. During each dialysis up to two or three litres of water can be removed by ultrafiltration which can compensate for excess fluid intake. In two-thirds of dialysis patients, control of water and sodium balance will maintain a normal or near normal blood pressure while the remainder will in addition require antihypertensive drugs. Oral supplements of iron, B and C vitamins and folic acid are required. The administration of aluminium hydroxide is usually necessary to control the serum phosphorus and 1α cholecalciferol may be indicated. The use of these two agents is discussed more fully in Chapter 10. Bilateral nephrectomy is required in a few patients. The indications are uncontrollable hypertension, active pyelonephritis, and polycystic kidneys which are very large or are associated with severe pain or bleeding.

Home haemodialysis

Two-thirds of patients in the United Kingdom dialyse at home although the number is much smaller in other countries. Almost all dialysis patients are suitable medically and the main limiting factor is the need for a helper. This is usually the spouse but can be a relative or close friend. Self dialysis without a helper is possible but seldom satisfactory. Installation of the machine can be accomplished by a room conversion or use of a prefabricated cabin in the garden; otherwise re-housing is required. Thorough training by a good teacher is important. This is usually done by a senior nurse during a period of six to eight weeks. Cannulation is the most important skill which must be learned. Home dialysis carries the advantage of lower costs, being not much more than half that of dialysis in hospital. Of greater importance to the patient are the advantages of increased flexibility of the timing of dialysis, the encouragement of a more self-reliant attitude and the ability of the patient to take advantage of holiday dialysis facilities. Avoidance of prolonged and frequent travelling is of great help to the patient who lives at a distance from the hospital unit. Dialysis in the home should be the aim for all patients, with hospital treatment reserved for the minority in whom home treatment is impossible.

Peritoneal dialysis

This technique dates from the early 1950's but has only been in large scale use since the mid 1960's. Its usefulness results from the presence of a large surface area of peritoneum, between one and two square metres in the adult. The capillaries within the peritoneal membrane are separated from the cavity only by a single layer of mesothelium. This has a slightly greater permeability than Cuprophan and therefore the advantage of better dialysis of larger molecule uraemic toxins but the disadvantage of causing protein loss. While widely used for short-term dialysis, the technique has had, until the late 1970's, a very limited long-term role, accounting for less than two per cent of long-term dialyses. The introduction of continuous ambulatory peritoneal dialysis (CAPD) by Popovich in 1976 with subsequent technical improvements by Oreopoulos in 1977 is considerably increasing the role of peritoneal dialysis. Following the insertion of a permanent peritoneal catheter, the patient can be trained in the technique during a period of one to two weeks. Sterile dialysis fluid from a two-litre plastic bag is run in through the catheter. The plastic bag and connecting tubing are then carried in a cloth purse or other receptacle wrapped round the waist. Several hours later, the plastic bag is laid on the floor and the dialysate drained out by gravity. At this point the bag is disconnected, a new one attached and the next cycle begins. The patient usually carries out four cycles every 24 hours, seven days per week. Considerable quantities of extra fluid can be removed by the osmotic effect of a high dextrose concentration in the dialysis fluid. This enables the patient to drink with relative freedom. Protein loss in the dialysis fluid is usually less than 10 g per day and with a free protein intake, depletion should not occur.

Choice of method

Haemodialysis is of proven value for periods of time exceeding ten years, and will continue to be the mainstay of dialysis therapy for some time. However, if longer term experience with CAPD bears out the early promise, this approach will come to be used more and more. In the initial selection, the presence of widespread vascular disease can lead to difficulty in obtaining vessel access and in such patients CAPD may be preferred. On the other hand, previous abdominal surgery with resultant adhesions is likely to lead to unsatisfactory CAPD. Reasonable intelligence and the willingness to adhere to a very careful technique are important to avoid the introduction of infection in CAPD. This is the main limiting factor on the number of suitable patients. Once treatment has started, haemodialysis has the advantage of being limited to three sessions per week while CAPD is a constant process, consuming two to three hours each day. Early experience with CAPD has shown smoother and better biochemical control than with haemodialysis, higher haemoglobin levels and improved well-being. Also the greater freedom with diet and fluid intake is appreciated by the patient. In conclusion, neither haemodialysis nor CAPD is ideal but the fact that there is now a choice goes some way to improve the lifestyle of the renal failure patient.

COMPLICATIONS OF DIALYSIS

The complications can be separated into those associated with the continuing presence of the renal failure and those directly resulting from the dialysis procedure itself.

Complications of renal failure

The complications most frequently encountered are:

Hypertension
Cardiac failure
Vascular disease
Anaemia
Depression
Sexual problems
Infection
Osteodystrophy
Neuropathy

Hypertension is usually sodium dependent and can be controlled by sodium and water restriction in the diet and their removal during dialysis. About one-third of patients remain hypertensive despite correction of sodium excess and require drug therapy. A beta blocker with the addition, if necessary, of a vasodilator such as hydralazine will usually give satisfactory control. In a few patients, poorly controlled blood pressure is associated with very high plasma renin levels and in these patients bilateral nephrectomy may be required.

Cardiac failure is a common complication with several causes contributing, in particular hypertension, anaemia, sodium retention and ischaemic heart disease. The avoidance of hypertension and sodium excess are therefore very important to maintain well-being and avoid premature death from cardiac failure.

Vascular disease occurs prematurely in many dialysis patients, and is due at least in part to the presence of hypertension and hyperlipidaemia. The latter occurs in at least one-third of patients mainly in the form of an elevated serum triglyceride. The clinical manifestations of the vascular disease follow the usual pattern of ischaemic heart disease, cerebrovascular accidents and peripheral vascular disease. There is no evidence that the dialysis procedure itself accelerates the process. Repeated thrombosis of vascular grafts may occur although AV fistulae are rarely affected.

Anaemia is almost always present with a haemoglobin usually between 7 and 10 g/100 ml, although a few patients can maintain a near normal value. Iron deficiency may be an aggravating factor and routine oral iron supplements are indicated. In a few patients the haemoglobin falls to a level at which the symptoms of dyspnoea and tiredness become unacceptable and periodic blood transfusion is required. This commonly happens after bilateral nephrectomy.

Depression is a common problem and is often precipitated by one of the complications of dialysis, such as loss of vessel access. Resolution of the complication will usually rapidly improve the patient's mood but antidepressant drugs may be of temporary value. Support from the family and hospital staff are essential components in the care of the dialysis patient.

Sexual problems are common but because the patient is often too embarrassed to discuss them, they may be overlooked. These include infertility in both sexes, impotence in the male and failure to achieve orgasm in the female. Discussion and advice can relieve some of the tension associated with these problems although the problems themselves cannot be resolved.

The remaining complications listed, infection, osteodystrophy and neuropathy, are discussed in Chapter 10.

Dialysis-associated complications

The more common problems associated with haemodialysis are:

Hypotension
Disequilibrium
Air embolism
Thrombosis of vessel access

Hypotension is usually due to excessive or too rapid fluid removal and can be rapidly corrected by an infusion of saline. Disequilibrium is rare except in the patient whose blood urea is rapidly lowered from a high level, as could occur during the first dialysis. It is due to cerebral oedema which results from the establishment of an osmotic gradient created by the slow removal of urea across the blood–brain barrier and the usual presentation is with convulsions. Air embolism will only occur if there is misuse or failure of the monitoring system. Loss of vessel access from thrombosis is discussed on page 208.

The most important complication of CAPD is peritonitis. The incidence can be lessened by well-designed equipment and careful attention to sterile technique when changing the bags and tubing. The incidence varies from one episode per eight patient months to one per 24 patient months depending on the technique and experience of the staff. The first evidence of peritonitis is cloudiness of the dialysis effluent and if intraperitoneal broad spectrum antibiotic therapy is started at this stage, resolution usually occurs within a few days. If untreated, clinical signs of peritonitis will develop and recovery will be much slower. Some patients eventually have to be transferred to haemodialysis because of repeated episodes of peritonitis. Blockage of the catheter by fibrin may occur but this will usually resolve with addition of heparin to the dialysate. Finally hypotension may occur as with haemodialysis due to excess sodium and water removal.

CAUSES OF DEATH

Disease of the cardiovascular system accounts for about 55 per cent of deaths in haemodialysis patients. Within this group, cardiac failure and strokes are the commonest individual causes. The high frequency of cardiovascular deaths reflects the effects of hypertension, anaemia and hyperlipidaemia. Infections account for 15 per cent of deaths resulting from these patients' impaired immune response. Less common causes are malignant disease (three per cent) and refusal to continue treatment (two per cent).

SURVIVAL AND REHABILITATION

The multinational statistics available through the European Dialysis and Transplant Association (EDTA) show that about 55 per cent of hospital haemodialysis patients survive for five years while the comparable figure for home dialysis is about 75 per cent. This difference is mainly the result of selection in that patients chosen for home dialysis tend to be fitter and more motivated.

Figure 11.1 shows that middle-aged patients undergoing dialysis and transplantation have a similar or better survival than patients of similar age with some of the more common potentially fatal diseases.

The rehabilitation of dialysis patients is surprisingly good considering the time spent with the procedure itself and the suboptimal state of health which often exists. Overall, about 35 per cent work full-time and 25 per cent part-time. Less than 15 per cent are unfit to work while the remaining 25 per cent have been unable to find suitable employment. Thus the admittedly crude assessment provided by rehabilitation rates shows that dialysis can not only maintain life but restore a reasonable degree of well-being to most patients.

THE FUTURE

Haemodialysis technology will continue to develop rapidly but the main benefits of this will be more portable machines with increased reliability and ease of operation. It is unlikely that dialysis times can be shortened to much less than the present minimum of 12 hours per week. Improved materials and technique will further reduce the incidence of peritonitis in CAPD patients leading to increased popularity of this method. Of considerable benefit would be the

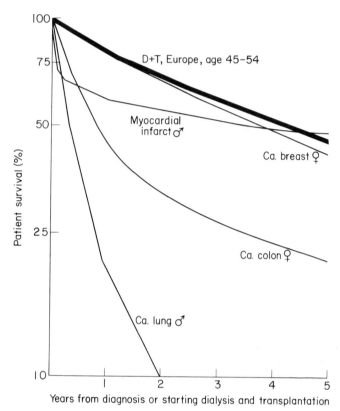

FIG. 11.1 This graph shows the percentage patient survival in a group of patients aged 45–54 years who were treated by a combination of dialysis and transplantation compared to patients of similar age with other potentially fatal diseases. *Proceedings of the European Dialysis and Transplantation Association* (1978) **15**, 22.

introduction of a preparation of erythropoietin as anaemia plays a major role in the symptomatology of the dialysis patient. Despite these advances, it is likely that dialysis will become more and more a temporary method of treatment for the patient awaiting transplantation.

POINTS OF EMPHASIS

● Most patients under 5 and over 70 are not suitable for dialysis.

● In suitable patients, dialysis is indicated before the onset of serious uraemic complications, usually when the creatinine clearance has fallen to about 5 ml/minute.

● AV fistula formation is the best long-term method for vessel access but an AV shunt has the advantage of immediate availability for use.

● Home haemodialysis is preferred because it is cheaper and allows a more flexible life stlye.

● CAPD usually gives better biochemical control and superior well-being compared with haemodialysis but has the disadvantage of predisposition to peritonitis.

● Hypertension can usually be controlled by dietary restriction and removal during dialysis of sodium. In about one-third of patients, drug therapy remains necessary and occasionally bilateral nephrectomy is required.

● Vascular disease occurs prematurely and accounts for about half of the deaths in dialysis patients.

● Anaemia is responsible for many of the symptoms but regular blood transfusion is not usually required unless the patient has undergone bilateral nephrectomy.

● Patients should be encouraged to discuss any sexual problems or episodes of depression.

● Common haemodialysis-associated problems are hypotension, disequilibrium, air embolism and thrombosis of vessel access.

● The five year survival for home haemodialysis is about 75 per cent.

CHAPTER 12

Renal transplantation

INTRODUCTION

Transplantation has the important advantage in comparison with dialysis, of being able to restore a degree of health close to or virtually indistinguishable from normal. It also removes the constraints of such things as diet, fluid intake and travel which the dialysis patient has to suffer. A third advantage is the much lower cost, less than 30 per cent of the cost of hospital haemodialysis, over a time scale of five years. The disadvantages in the past have been a high failure rate requiring return to dialysis and an increased mortality in the short term although recent experience suggests that a considerable improvement is taking place in both patient and graft survival.

THE DONOR

Live donor

Although accounting for only 10 per cent of transplants in Europe, the live donor transplant has the advantage of a higher success rate, avoidance of a long waiting period on dialysis, and immediate graft function. The disadvantage is the small but real risk of serious operative or postoperative complications in the donor. Only siblings or parents with at least one haplotype in common with the recipient should be considered as donors.

Cadaver donor

Only patients with brain death who are being maintained on a mechanical ventilator can be considered as kidney donors. The most common causes of such irreversible brain damage are head injury and subrarachnoid haemorrhage, but others include primary intracranial tumours and hypoxic damage. Contraindications to kidney donation are:

Age below 5 or over 60 years.
Malignant disease (except primary intracranial tumours).
Overwhelming infection.
Moderate or severe hypertension.
Renal disease.
Anuria or oliguria unresponsive to therapy.

The age criteria are not rigid and only intended as a guide.

Brain death should be established on two occasions with an interval of a few hours or longer using the following clinical tests:

1. *No spontaneous respiration for five minutes*
   (on intratracheal O_2 ($Pa CO_2$ >45 mmHg))
2. *No brain stem reflexes.*
   No light reflex (pupils fixed).
   No corneal reflex.
   No gag reflex.
   No caloric (oculovestibular) reflex.
   No motor responses in the face following painful stimuli.

Written consent from a close relative should be obtained unless the donor possessed a signed donor card. Thereafter attention must be paid to maintaining good renal perfusion by such measures as intravenous fluids and mannitol and the use of dopamine in the presence of oliguria. Pretreatment with such drugs as heparin, prednisolone and phenoxybenzamine shortly before cessation of ventilation may be beneficial. Ideally the nephrectomy procedure should be carried out or at least initiated while ventilation is maintained. If this is not possible, the kidneys should be removed immediately after cardiac arrest although viable kidneys can be obtained if removed within 45 minutes. This interval is the warm ischaemic time. Either before or after removal, the kidneys are perfused with a chilled solution and, once cooled, they will remain fully viable for up to 24 hours if stored in ice (the cold ischaemic time), or for two to three days if perfused in a machine.

PREPARATION OF THE RECIPIENT

Patient selection

Most dialysis patients between the ages of 5 and 60 years are suitable for transplantation; patients over 60 years are usually excluded since mortality rises with age. Oxalosis is the only cause of renal failure which contraindicates transplantation although special problems exist with some others such as diabetes mellitus, obstructive uropathy and renal tumours.

General assessment

Before proceeding to transplantation, any infection should be eradicated and the blood pressure controlled. Endoscopy should be performed and if a peptic ulcer is present, it should be treated by cimetidine or surgery.

Preliminary operations

Bilateral nephrectomy is indicated in the presence of uncontrollable hypertension, chronic pyelonephritis with active renal infection and very large polycystic kidneys. These indications taken together occur in only a small percentage of dialysis patients. Nephrectomy is best carried out electively prior to transplantation although the two operations can be combined. Splenectomy may improve graft survival but the benefit is not sufficient to justify the operation.

Preoperative preparation

Only limited time is available in cadaver transplantation. Dialysis should be carried out unless completed within the previous 24 hours and a blood transfusion given if the haematocrit is less than 25 per cent.

MATCHING FOR HLA

The histocompatibility complex (HLA complex) on chromosome 6 contains four loci, A, B, C and D. At each locus there are two antigens, one inherited from each parent. So far the C locus has not been shown to have much relevance to transplantation. More than 20 antigens have been defined at the A locus and more than 40 at the B locus with serological methods using lymphocyte preparations from peripheral blood, lymph nodes or spleen. The D locus was initially defined using mixed lymphocyte culture (MLC) and recently serological methods have been used with the demonstration so far of 10 antigens. These serologically defined antigens are termed DR as they may not be identical although closely related to the D locus antigens as demonstrated by MLC. The benefit of matching at the A, B and D loci has been unequivocally demonstrated in live donor transplantation. Thus the success rate when both haplotypes are shared by donor and recipient is significantly better than when only one is shared. There is less certainty of the influence of HLA matching in cadaver transplantation. The bulk of evidence now suggests that when three or four of the A and B locus antigens or both the DR antigens are shared, the success rate is higher than with poorer degrees of match. There is not, however, unanimity of opinion on this point. Once the best possible match has been chosen on the basis of the HLA antigens, a negative cross-match must be demonstrated between the T lymphocytes of the donor and the recipient's serum. As a result of the large number of HLA antigens and therefore very large number of possible HLA types in the population, a large pool of potential recipients must be available to allow the transplantation of well-matched kidneys. Thus national and international organ sharing schemes have been established with efficient methods of transporting kidneys from one centre to another. The British scheme, UK Transplant, has the names of more than 1000 patients within its computer memory at any one time.

TRANSPLANT OPERATION

Surgical technique

The donor kidney is placed in either the right or left iliac fossa.

The first of the three anastomoses is between the donor renal vein and the recipient external iliac vein. Next the donor artery is joined end-to-side to the external iliac artery or end-to-end to the anterior branch of the internal iliac artery. The final part of the operation consists of implantation of the ureter into the bladder.

Anaesthesia

There are three points of particular importance. Firstly, severe anaemia makes the avoidance of hypoxia even more essential than usual. Secondly, the drugs used and their dose should be chosen with care to avoid prolonged effects from drugs which are normally rapidly excreted. Thirdly, there is a high incidence of ventilatory inadequacy following anaesthesia in renal failure. Two factors may be involved, prolonged curarisation or re-curarisation, and the depressant effect of narcotics. Pancuronium is a useful muscle relaxant as it is partly excreted in the bile and the dose of narcotics should be limited as much as possible.

IMMUNOSUPPRESSION

Prednisolone and azathioprine form the mainstay of therapy.

Prednisolone

There is increasing evidence that a relatively low dose is as effective as a much higher one. A typical 'low dose' regime consists of 20 mg per day for three months followed by progressive reduction to a maintenance level of 7·5–15 mg per day. Administration of this maintenance dose on alternate days, i.e. 15–30 mg, may reduce the incidence of side-effects. Most evidence suggests that prednisolone must be continued even in the long term except with highly compatible grafts. The much larger doses used to treat rejection are discussed below. Steroid side-effects are discussed with the other complications of transplantation.

Azathioprine

This drug is given in a single daily dose of 1–3 mg/kg. The main side-effect is marrow depression which is reversible with reduction of the dose. There is increasing evidence that many grafts will continue to function well if azathioprine is discontinued after a few months. It is not, however, possible to predict in whom continuation of azathioprine is necessary and therefore it should only be stopped if side-effects such as leucopenia arise.

Antilymphocyte globulin (ALG)

This material is effective in many animal experiments but is not of proven value in human renal transplantation.

Cyclosporin A

This new drug is a highly effective immunosuppressive agent but is nephrotoxic and may carry a high risk of development of lymphomas. Further evaluation is needed.

Other methods

Radiotherapy and lymphocyte drainage through the thoracic duct have been abandoned.

POST-OPERATIVE CARE

Immediate respiratory care

Awareness by the nursing staff of the possibility of ventilatory inadequacy is important. Muscle power can be simply assessed by requesting the patient to lift his head or squeeze the examiner's fingers. Poor muscle power provides a warning that the depth and rate of respiration should be closely observed. Inadequate reversal of neuromuscular blocking agents can be corrected by neostigmine and persistence of narcotic effect can be abolished by naloxone. Oxygen should be given for the first few hours to avoid hypoxia.

General management

If the kidney does not function immediately, haemodialysis is continued during the oliguric phase with control of fluid and dietary intake. With long warm ischaemic times the onset of function may be delayed for two to three weeks. Measures to prevent infection are important in view of the increased susceptibility induced by the uraemic state and immunosuppressive drugs. These should include the use of a single cubicle (but not necessarily complete isolation), careful aseptic techniques and frequent bacteriological monitoring of the patient and the environment.

Surveillance and investigations

If there is an initial oliguric period, serial isotope scans using ^{99m}Technetium or ^{99m}Technetium—DTPA provide a sensitive guide to both renal artery thrombosis and acute rejection. Prior to discharge, endoscopy should be performed in view of the high incidence of peptic ulcer and probable aggravating effect of steroids. Severe inflammation, erosions or a peptic ulcer are indications for cimetidine and a further examination later. Following discharge, visits should be every day or two at first to enable rejection to be detected early. The interval between visits can then be gradually increased up to three months by the end of the first year. Apart from routine blood and urine tests, IVUs or Hippuran renograms should be carried out once or twice a year to detect the development of ureteric stenosis, and bone X-rays or isotope scans during the first three or four years to detect bone necrosis. Finally hepatitis Bs Ag testing should continue as long as the patient attends the transplant unit despite the decreased risk of hepatitis at this stage.

REJECTION

Rejection is by far the most common cause of graft failure, accounting for three-quarters of all failures. Four clinical types are recognised, hyperacute, accelerated, acute and chronic.

Hyperacute rejection

Within minutes or hours of completion of the vascular anastomosis, the kidney becomes blue and mottled. This is due to either ABO blood group incompatibility or circulating antibodies which react with the donor HLA antigens. If correct blood grouping and performance of a crossmatch between donor lymphocytes and recipient serum is carried out, this should not occur. It is irreversible and an indication for immediate transplant nephrectomy.

Accelerated rejection

This develops within one to four days of transplantation. It occurs in patients who have previously been exposed to HLA antigens possessed by the donor but in whom the serum used for the crossmatch test does not contain a significant titre of antibody. It is almost always irreversible.

Acute rejection

This, by far the most common type, occurs between one week and several months from the time of the transplant. Clinical signs are unreliable and the most useful diagnostic features are sudden weight gain, reduction in urine volume, rise in serum creatinine or fall in creatinine clearance. A percutaneous biopsy is relatively simple and safe and is useful for diagnostic and prognostic purposes where severe rejection is suspected. Treatment consists either of high dose oral steroids or intravenous infusions of prednisolone, the usual dose of the latter being one gram, often repeated two or three times on successive days. Intravenous doses of less than one gram would probably also be effective. Most rejection episodes will resolve with this therapy, but if more than one episode occurs within the first few weeks, later irreversible rejection is likely.

Chronic rejection

The initial presentation is often the insidious onset of proteinuria occurring more than three months, and often several years after transplantation. It is progressive although often only slowly, and not responsive to steroids, leading eventually to loss of the kidney. It presents in a similar manner to recurrence of glomerulonephritis but can usually be differentiated by biopsy.

Prevention of rejection

A careful crossmatch should prevent hyperacute rejection and to a certain extent the accelerated type if previous sera from the patient are used rather than only a current sample. Chronic rejection is too poorly understood for prevention to be effective. However, much can be done to reduce the incidence of acute rejection. HLA matching and the use of immunosuppressive drugs have already been discussed. A further preventive measure is blood transfusion. There is now substantial evidence that blood transfusion prior to transplantation substantially improves graft survival by decreasing the incidence of acute rejection. Several units are probably more effective than one and whole blood is probably more effective than leucocyte free blood. The mode of action of blood transfusion has not yet been fully explained.

COMPLICATIONS AFFECTING THE GRAFT

Vascular complications

Arterial thrombosis affects a few per cent of transplants and almost always leads to infarction and loss of the kidney. Venous thrombosis is uncommon and may present with ipsilateral leg swelling and heavy proteinuria. At a later stage, stenosis of the artery can occur, again in a few per cent of cases, presenting with hypertension. It can be treated surgically, although there is a high technical failure rate, or by dilatation of the stenosed segment using a balloon catheter.

Ureteric complications

Fistulae can develop from the bladder or lower end of ureter, the former usually from the site of the bladder incision. Ureteric fistulae usually result from a poor blood supply to the lower ureter with ischaemic necrosis. The presentation in both cases is sudden onset of severe pain, swelling of the subcutaneous tissues and fever. Radiology may help to localise the site of the leak, and immediate surgery is required. A later complication is stenosis of the lower end of the ureter which presents as a hydronephrosis and is corrected by excision of the stenosed segment and re-implantation of the ureter into the bladder.

Miscellaneous complications

A few per cent of kidneys are non-viable, usually due to ante-mortem hypotension or prolonged warm ischaemia. The initial ^{99m}Technetium scan will suggest this and biopsy can provide confirmation. Graft rupture is an uncommon but highly dangerous complication which will present with severe pain and signs of blood loss and will usually require nephrectomy. Peri-renal fluid collections usually consist of lymphoceles but can be due to abscess or haematoma. The ultrasound is very useful in diagnosis and localisation, enabling aspiration of lymphoceles to be performed safely. An abscess will require incision and drainage.

COMPLICATIONS AFFECTING THE PATIENT

Infection
    Bacterial
    Mycobacterial
    Fungal
    Viral
    Pneumocystis carinii
Gastrointestinal
    Peptic ulcer
    Acute pancreatitis
    Hepatic damage
    Perforation of colon
Diabetes mellitus
Bone necrosis
Tumours
Miscellaneous
    Obesity
    Hirsutism
    Moon face
    Acne
    Cataract
Cardiovascular
    Myocardial ischaemia
    Cardiac failure
    Hypertension
    Cerebrovascular disease
Hypercalcaemia

Infection

One-third of deaths after transplantation are due to infection and most of these occur in the first two years. There are a number of predisposing factors of which large doses of steroids are the most important. This fact strengthens the argument in favour of low dose steroids as discussed on page 222.

Bacteria account for two-thirds of infections, mainly in the urinary and respiratory tracts, wounds and vessel access areas. One quarter of transplant patients have an episode of septicaemia. Frequent bacteriological surveillance and effective antibiotic therapy are important.

Mycobacterial infection, in the form of tuberculosis, will occur in a few per cent of transplant patients in areas where this disease is still prevalent. Detection of the organism is difficult and false negative tuberculin skin tests occur. Therapy may need to be started when strong clinical suspicion exists and a good response can be expected.

Fungal infection is seen, on average, in five to ten per cent of patients although occasional reports quote a much higher figure. The fungi commonly encountered are *aspergilli*, mainly causing pneumonia but occasionally brain abscess, *Candida*, usually leading to oesophagitis and gastritis but sometimes becoming disseminated and more rarely *Cryptococcus* with pulmonary or CNS infection. The anti-fungal drugs available are amphotericin, flucytosine and several imidazoles including ketoconazole, miconazole and econazole. In most cases, an effective drug or combination of drugs can be found but as with all these opportunistic infections, the main problem is making the diagnosis early enough.

Viral infection is very common although often subclinical. The herpes group, in particular cytomegalovirus (CMV), predominate. CMV can occur as a primary infection, usually transmitted by the kidney, in those with no previous exposure, and much more often as reactivation of latent infection. The former is more serious, the main features being hepatitis and pneumonitis but both types can also precipitate acute rejection.

Pneumocystis carinii is a parasite which is rarely seen in normal practice but can cause pneumonitis in immunosuppressed patients. The typical features are an unproductive cough and progressive dyspnoea with hypoxia an early feature. The diagnosis rests on demonstration of the parasite in sections from lung biopsy although this procedure carries a high incidence of complications. High dose septrin, 12 tablets per day, is usually effective, with pentamidine as the second choice.

Gastrointestinal complications

Peptic ulcer or erosions occur in five to ten per cent of cases, and routine endoscopy should be performed. Acute lesions are more common and will usually heal with cimetidine. This is an important complication, since if undetected and bleeding occurs, the mortality is up to 50 per cent.

Diabetes mellitus

With high dose steroids, the majority of patients develop hyperglycaemia which usually settles as the dose is reduced, but a few patients require insulin or oral drugs. This complication substantially increases that risk of infection.

Bone necrosis

This occurs most often in the hips and is asymptomatic in almost half of patients. The incidence increases progressively with time, reaching over 30 per cent by five years. High dose steroids are again the main precipitating factor.

Tumours

The incidence is six per cent, 100 times greater than in the general population, with carcinoma of skin and lips and lymphomas the most common.

Cardiovascular complications

These cause a similar mortality to infection, accounting for one-third of deaths, but unlike infection are often late complications. Predisposing factors include hypertension, hyperlipidaemia and hyperglycaemia. Hypertension is important on its own account as it is common in the transplant patient. The patient's own diseased kidneys are the most common cause but stenosis of the transplant renal artery must not be overlooked.

Hypercalcaemia

Hyperparathyroidism is common in renal insufficiency and failure of the glands to involute following transplantation may lead to hypercalcaemia and sometimes the need for parathyroidectomy.

Most of the above complications are due mainly to steroid therapy. As steroids have been used in high dose in most centres until recently, the frequency of these complications should be seen in this context. The change to low dose steroids now taking place can be expected to reduce considerably the incidence of these complications.

RESULTS OF TRANSPLANTATION

Table 12.1 compares patient survival following transplantation with that on long term dialysis. Graft survival continues to be significantly better with living related donors than cadaver donors (Table 12.2) and the one year survival with an identical match sibling donor exceeds 90 per cent. Although patient survival on dialysis and after transplantation is similar, the quality of life after transplantation is greatly superior in both the standard of health and

TABLE 12.1   Patient survival following dialysis and transplantation (per cent).

	1 Year	2 Years	5 Years	10 Years
Hospital dialysis	86	75	54	39
Home dialysis	94	88	74	55
First live donor graft	86	81	69	59
First cadaver graft	76	69	56	44

TABLE 12.2   Survival of grafts from living and cadaver donors (per cent).

	1 Year	2 Years	3 Years
Living donor	73	68	64
Cadaver donor	53	47	44

freedom from restrictions on fluid intake and diet and the time-consuming dialysis itself. The transplanted patient can participate in most pastimes such as active sports and can have successful pregnancies, neither of which are possible on dialysis. For these reasons most patients, if given the choice, choose transplantation.

THE FUTURE

Transplantation is undergoing rapid change. After a rather stagnant period during most of the 1970's, substantial improvement is now taking place in both patient and graft survival. The improved patient survival is due largely to a lower incidence of infection resulting from more careful use of immunosuppressive drugs and in particular the use of low dose steroid regimes. The higher graft survival is almost entirely due to fewer rejection episodes. In turn this reduction in rejection follows the use of routine pre-transplant blood transfusion and also improving HLA matching techniques. Once the supply of cadaver donor kidneys has risen to approach the number required, transplantation will become firmly established as the treatment of choice for most patients with chronic renal failure.

POINTS OF EMPHASIS

● Successful renal transplantation offers a better quality of life than dialysis.

● Live donor transplant from a sibling or parent carries a higher success rate than cadaver donor transplant.

● Most dialysis patients are suitable for transplantation.

● Both live and cadaver transplants are more successful when there is a good HLA match.

● Prednisolone and azathioprine form the mainstay of immunosuppression.

● Low dose prednisolone is probably as effective and is much safer than a high dose regimen.

● Rejection accounts for three-quarters of graft failures.

- Most acute rejection episodes respond to high dose steroid therapy.

- Chronic rejection usually presents insidiously as proteinuria and is not steroid responsive.

- Blood transfusion prior to transplantation decreases the incidence of acute rejection.

- A third of deaths after transplantation are due to infection, mainly in the respiratory tract.

- Measures to prevent postoperative infection should include routine bacteriological monitoring of patient and environment.

- Routine postoperative endoscopy should be performed and any peptic ulcer or erosion treated with cimetidine.

- Tumours develop in 6 per cent of transplant patients.

- Patient survival following transplantation is similar to that on long-term dialysis.

CHAPTER 13

Drugs and the kidney

DRUGS CAUSING RENAL DYSFUNCTION

The kidney is particularly susceptible to damage caused by drugs because of its high blood flow, complex biochemical pathways and complicated structure. There are therefore a great number of ways in which drugs may affect the kidney, and an accurate drug history is important in any patient presenting with renal abnormalities.

Acute tubular necrosis (ATN)

Drugs capable of causing ATN are listed on page 164. Patients usually present with progressive increases in serum creatinine or oliguric acute renal failure. There may be few symptoms until renal failure is well advanced (see Chapter 9). The exact mechanism by which drugs cause ATN remains obscure. One hypothesis is that they cause necrosis of the proximal tubular cells. As a result, the concentration of sodium in the tubular fluid delivered to the distal convoluted cells is high and blood flow to their glomeruli is reduced by an unidentified tubulo-glomerular feedback.

Once the offending drug has been withdrawn, recovery of renal function is the rule providing that the patient is adequately supported during the period of failure (see Chapter 9). Some nephrotoxins such as paracetamol may cause lethal lesions in other organs from which the patient may die. If the kidney alone is involved, then failure to recover is exceptional.

Acute interstitial nephritis (AIN)

AIN may develop in patients treated with the following drugs:

Penicillin
Methicillin
Ampicillin
Carbenicillin
Rifampicin
Sulphonamides
Phenobarbitone
Phenindione
Allopurinol
Azathioprine

Only a fraction of patients treated by any particular drug will develop AIN, and some drugs are incriminated on the basis of a single case report.

The patient usually develops a fever, rash, arthralgia, eosinophilia, haematuria which is usually microscopic, mild proteinuria and renal failure. Renal biopsy reveals that the glomeruli appear normal but that the interstitium is grossly expanded by oedema and infiltrated with polymorph neutrophils and eosinophils. The illness usually resolves spontaneously within two or three weeks of stopping the offending drug, but a degree of renal failure may persist in the more severe reactions. For this reason steroids have been used to reduce the acute inflammatory reaction within the kidney with anecdotal success. Dialysis may be necessary to support the patient during the acute stage.

Chronic interstitial nephritis

Analgesic nephropathy has been discussed in Chapter 4. Tablets containing aspirin, phenacetin or paracetamol should be avoided in patients with chronic interstitial nephritis.

Renal tubular disorders

Renal tubular acidosis may occur in patients treated with acetazolamide, amphotericin or outdated tetracycline. Amphotericin, carbenicillin and other penicillins given in large doses may cause hypokalaemic alkalosis. Diabetes insipidus occurs in some patients treated with lithium, demeclocycline and methoxyflurane. The latter may cause irreversible renal failure as well. For clinical details see Chapter 5.

Glomerulitis

This is caused by some drugs as part of a generalised arteritis of small vessels. It may be difficult to prove a causal relationship as the clinical picture is often complicated and the drug has usually been started after the patient had developed symptoms which may subsequently be interpreted as part of a multisystem disease. Sulphonamides are the most commonly implicated drugs. The clinical picture is one of renal failure with proteinuria developing in a patient with evidence of involvement of other systems. A focal proliferative or crescentic nephritis is usually found on biopsy.

The nephrotic syndrome

This may develop in patients treated with gold, penicillamine or troxidone (see Chapter 6).

Obstruction

Obstruction may occur as a result of retroperitoneal fibrosis caused by methysergide, which is now rarely used because of this complication. Urate crystals may be deposited in the tubules early in the treatment of myeloproliferative disorders. This can usually be prevented by starting allopurinol before cytotoxic therapy. Ureteric obstruction may be caused by a papilla sloughed as a result of papillary necrosis following long term analgesic abuse.

DRUGS AGGRAVATING URAEMIA

Drugs which provoke catabolism cause a rise in blood urea. Steroids and tetracyclines are the most commonly used offenders. Tetracyclines, with the exception of doxycycline, inhibit the anabolism of amino acids to protein and thus encourage their degradation to urea. The rise in urea may induce uraemic symptoms and provoke vomiting which may lead to hypovolaemia and a reduction in renal function. Therefore, all tetracyclines, with the exception of doxycycline, should be avoided in patients with renal failure. Steroids also promote a rise in the urea but cause some salt and water retention; therefore, dehydration and reduction of renal function are much less common than with the tetracycline group.

DRUG THERAPY IN RENAL FAILURE

It is a sound rule, but not easy to follow, that no drug should ever be given to any patient unnecessarily. However, if the patient has renal failure, this rule should be strictly adhered to because many drugs or their major metabolites are excreted by the kidney and have to be given in reduced dosages or at longer intervals. Not surprisingly, drug reactions are three times more common in patients with renal failure than in those with normal renal function. If there is a clear indication for drug therapy, a drug which is not excreted by the kidney should be chosen if possible (Table 13.1). Most drugs, even if entirely excreted by the kidney, can be given at their usual dosage until the patient's creatinine clearance falls below 25 ml per minute. Thereafter, it is important to adjust the dose according to renal function which may be most conveniently assessed by measuring the creatinine clearance. The loading dose of a drug, i.e. that dose required to reach the desired concentration in the extracellular fluid, is unchanged. Subsequent doses of a drug entirely excreted by the kidney should be adjusted by the following formula:

$$\text{Adjusted dose} = \text{Normal dose} \times \frac{\text{Patient's creatinine clearance}}{\text{Normal creatinine clearance}}$$

If the drug is partially metabolised and partially excreted unchanged in the kidney, then the formula is more complex:

$$\text{Adjusted dose} = f(kf - 1) + 1$$

Where f = fraction of the drug normally excreted by the kidney

and k $= \dfrac{\text{Patient's creatinine clearance}}{\text{Normal creatinine clearance}}$

Dosage schedules for most of the more common drugs have been worked out for varying degrees of renal failure and these can be consulted. If possible, plasma concentration of the drug should be

TABLE 13.1 Drug therapy in renal failure.

Largely excreted by non-renal routes: dose unaltered

Clindamycin	Opiates
Lincomycin	Diazepam
Erythromycin	Short acting barbiturates
Doxycycline	Phenothiazines
Metronidazole	Azathioprine
Isoniazid	Cyclophosphamide
Rifampicin	Warfarin
Phenylbutazone	Heparin
Indomethacin	Digitoxin
Prednisolone	Phenytoin
Chlorpropamide	

Excreted by kidney but toxic/therapeutic level ratio high

Penicillins	Allopurinol
Cephaloridine	Aspirin
Cefazolin	

Excreted by renal (per cent) and non-renal route

Carbenicillin	60
Cephalothin	60
Tetracycline	45
Phenformin	70
Digoxin	80 (Not dialysable)

Excreted by kidney with low toxic/therapeutic ratio

Gentamicin and all aminoglycosides
Ethambutol
5-Fluorocytosine
Phenobarbitone

Drugs metabolised but toxic metabolites excreted by kidney

Chloramphenicol
Nalidixic acid

measured serially to correct any error and the patient should be seen frequently so that complications can be detected as early as possible. If these rules are observed, almost any drug can be given to a patient with renal failure.

Antibiotics and renal failure

Infection is particularly common in patients with acute renal failure and it is important to be able to treat it safely. *The penicillins*, including carbenicillin, are largely excreted unchanged by the kidney, but the difference between therapeutic and toxic levels is so large that they can be used in normal doses except when very large doses are required as in the treatment of infective endocarditis. The signs of penicillin overdosage are impairment of the level of consciousness, myoclonic twitching and convulsions. Furthermore, very large doses of any penicillin also give a large amount of sodium which may be dangerous if the patient is unable to excrete the extra load.

The aminoglycosides are also excreted by the kidney and the difference between therapeutic and toxic levels is much less than that of penicillin. Therefore, the dose should be reduced and blood levels checked frequently. The major toxic effects are nerve deafness and vertigo, which are not reversible, and renal failure, which is. Gentamicin is frequently used in patients with acute tubular necrosis and does not appear to impair recovery of renal function.

Of *the cephalosporins*, cephaloridine is entirely eliminated by the kidney and causes tubular damage particularly if given with an aminoglycoside or a loop diuretic. It should not be used in patients with renal failure. Cephalothin is both excreted unchanged by the kidney and esterified in the liver. It is less nephrotoxic and can be given safely to patients with renal failure although the dose should be reduced. The newer cephalosporins also appear to be safe.

Nitrofurantoin is usually given for the treatment of urinary tract infections because it is concentrated in the urine. This no longer happens when the creatinine clearance falls below 50 ml per minute and it should not be used in these patients.

Sulphonamides are excreted by the kidney and the dose should be reduced when the patient's creatinine clearance falls below 25 ml per minute. This group of drugs is capable of causing a wide variety of reactions harmful to the kidney (see above) and therefore their use should be restricted in patients with renal failure.

Tetracyclines (exept doxycycline), *nalidixic acid and chloramphenicol* should all be avoided in patients with renal failure, the latter two because their major metabolites are toxic and excreted by the kidney.

Anti-tuberculosis therapy in uraemic patients

Patients with renal failure have depressed cellular immunity and might be expected to have a higher incidence of tuberculosis. This has never been substantiated, but patients with renal failure who develop tuberculosis do pose a difficult clinical problem. Fortunately, isoniazid and rifampicin are mostly metabolised in the liver and can be given in normal doses to patients with renal failure. However, ethambutol and para-aminosalicylic acid are largely excreted unchanged by the kidney and therefore the dose has to be reduced. Of the second line drugs, pyrazinamide and ethionamide may be given in normal doses.

Glycosides

Digoxin is 80 per cent excreted by the kidney but is not removed by haemodialysis. Therefore, the dose should be reduced in patients with renal failure and the serum level checked frequently. Digitoxin is metabolised by the liver and can be used in normal doses. However, most doctors are less familiar with this preparation and the assay to measure the serum concentration is not generally available, so digoxin continues to be used.

The dose of many drugs is normally titrated according to their biological effect. Common examples are hypotensive drugs, diuretics, analgesics, hypoglycaemic agents and soporifics. The actual dose given to any particular patient with renal failure may be judged according to the effect desired provided this does not produce unacceptable side effects. Thus the presence of renal failure does not alter the normal clinical practice with these groups of drugs, but frequent clinical assessment of the patient is required.

POINTS OF EMPHASIS

● The kidney is particularly susceptible to drug damage.

● A variety of drugs may produce various renal tubular disorders, ATN, acute or chronic interstitial nephritis, glomerulitis, nephrotic syndrome or obstruction.

● Drug reactions occur three times more often in patients with renal failure.

● Tetracyclines (except doxycycline), nalidixic acid and chloramphenicol should be avoided in renal failure.

● Apply the following general principles in considering the use of drugs in renal failure:

1. Only treat if there is a clear clinical indication.

2. Choose a drug which is not excreted by the kidney. If this is not available, choose a drug with a shorter half-life, e.g. tolbutamide, rather than chlorpropamide.

3. Consult a nomogram to determine the recommended dose of the drug for a particular patient's renal function.

4. If possible, measure the plasma drug concentration at frequent intervals.

5. Watch the patient carefully for the development of side-effects.

6. Stop the drug as soon as practical.

CHAPTER 14

Urological problems of the kidney

SURGICAL ASPECTS OF CONGENITAL RENAL ABNORMALITY

These are described in Chapter 3. In general, it is unhelpful to try surgical procedures to correct abnormal X-ray appearances but surgery may be helpful to relieve obstruction, e.g. ureteric obstruction in association with a horse-shoe kidney.

RENAL INJURY

Renal injuries may be blunt or sharp, major or minor.

Major renal injury

Major renal injury occurs when there is disruption of one of the large vessels resulting in significant blood loss. Such a patient is shocked and initial treatment consists of securing the airway and replacing lost blood volume. If the patient's condition permits, it is extremely helpful to have an arteriogram to try to define which vessel is involved. The safe approach is to explore surgically the renal area and to remove the injured kidney tying off the bleeding vessel. It is essential, however, to confirm that there is a normal kidney on the other side, since in an emergency situation, this can sometimes be overlooked. Usually an exploratory operation is combined with a laparotomy to exclude other intra-abdominal injury. If however a renal injury is unsuspected but a retroperitoneal haematoma is discovered during the course of a laparotomy for intraperitoneal haemorrhage then the correct course of action is to leave the haematoma alone and to close the abdomen after stopping any bleeding from liver or spleen. The renal injury may then be defined by intravenous urography and if necessary arteriography. If the area of kidney damage has been defined by preoperative arteriography it is sometimes possible to evacuate the haematoma and repair the injured vessel. Most renal injuries seen in this country are caused by blunt trauma following road traffic accidents.

Penetrating injury

Any penetrating stab wound should be explored surgically: occasionally these will enter the kidney and cause massive blood loss. It is worth noting that haemorrhage following stab wounds can be delayed and the patient's initial good condition does not alter the surgical rule that all stab wounds should be explored.

Minor trauma

A number of patients present with mild trauma, e.g. haematuria following a rugby match injury. In these cases an intravenous urogram will usually demonstrate normal anatomy or occasionally a peri-renal haematoma. Treatment is conservative.

RENAL OBSTRUCTION (Fig. 14.1)

Calyceal obstruction

This is usually secondary to stenosis of the calyceal neck following fibrosis from tuberculosis. Primary obstruction may be consequent upon a neuromuscular defect. The upper calyx is sometimes said to become obstructed because of vessels crossing the neck of the calyx.

Pelviureteric junction obstruction

Pelvic hydronephrosis is a congenital abnormality, usually bilateral, where there is obstruction to the passage of urine at the pelviureteric junction. The aetiology is either due to a muscular deficiency in the

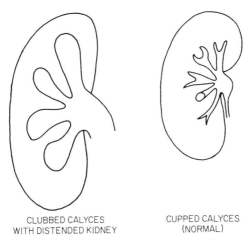

CLUBBED CALYCES
WITH DISTENDED KIDNEY

CUPPED CALYCES
(NORMAL)

FIG. 14.1   The effect of obstruction on renal anatomy.

last part of the renal pelvis and the first part of the ureter or because of a lower pole renal artery crossing and kinking the ureter.

CLINICAL PRESENTATION

Babies may present with failure to thrive because of renal failure; sometimes there is a prominent abdominal mass. In older children there can be loin pain often associated with symptoms of urinary infection. In adults the presentation is usually loin pain, particularly after a fluid load.

DIAGNOSIS

The diagnosis is made by intravenous urography. It is usually wise to check that the rest of the ureter is normal by retrograde urography before committing the patient to operation.

TREATMENT

Operation is usually required to free the pelviureteric junction from the adhesions and to excise the deranged segment of ureter

(Anderson Hynes pyeloplasty). If the obstruction is caused by a crossing vessel, it is sometimes possible to reposition the vessel without having to excise any ureter. Bilateral pelviureteric junction obstruction is common and the contralateral kidney should always be carefully assessed.

URINARY TRACT STONE

Surgical treatment

Patients presenting with renal colic are usually in acute pain (Chapter 2). The doctor's first concern is to relieve this pain. Because these patients are usually aged 30–40 pain sensation has not been dulled by old age and relief is often only obtained with large doses of narcotic analgesics. It is wise therefore to confirm the diagnosis by seeing the size of the stone on a plain X-ray and confirming the degree of obstruction by IVU. A small proportion of uric acid calculi are radiolucent; obstruction without an obvious stone on the plain film does not exclude stones. In such cases a retrograde pyelogram may demonstrate a lucent calculus although the same information can often be obtained by delayed films of the intravenous urogram series.

INDICATIONS FOR OPERATION

1. Complete or severe partial obstruction for more than six weeks without any progress of the stone down the ureter.
2. Infection or pus above the stone is a surgical emergency (compare acute appendicitis) and operation to relieve obstruction and drain pus should be performed immediately. Such a patient is ill, febrile and has severe loin pain and tenderness in addition to a previous history of ureteric colic. This situation may occur after failed instrumentation to remove a ureteric stone.
3. Stones less than 0·5 cm have an 80 per cent chance of being passed. Larger stones usually require operative removal although if a large stone is obviously progressing down the ureter on a series of plain films operation may be deferred.
4. Severe pain such that analgesic addiction becomes a possibility is an indication for operation.
5. Obstruction in a single kidney causing uraemia.

6. If the stone or stones are causing a deterioration in renal function, particularly in patients with chronic renal failure.

SURGERY TO REMOVE STONES

Pyelolithotomy and ureterolithotomy

Stones in the kidney or upper two-thirds of the ureter are most satisfactorily removed at open operation. Stones in the kidney are removed through a loin incision. Sometimes, in order to remove a large kidney stone, it is necessary to clamp the renal artery and cool the kidney (to preserve renal function). Most kidney stones are removed by way of incision in the renal pelvis (pyelolithotomy). Ureteric stones are usually approached through an anterior abdominal incision.

Ureteric basket

Stones in the lower one-third of the ureter may be removed using a ureteric basket. This is an expanding wire cage which is passed up the ureter by way of a cystoscope. This technique is dangerous if the stone is too large or too high up the ureter.

Medical treatment

Once the patient's symptoms have been dealt with investigations are needed to determine the cause of stone formation. It should be remembered that stone formation starts at home when the patient is active and investigations of the recumbent postoperative patient are of questionable value.

INCIDENCE

A recent whole population survey of Cumbernauld (near Glasgow) showed that four per cent of the population had urinary tract stones (four per cent prevalence). In some North American cities, the incidence (life time incidence) is thought to approach 12 per cent.

Types of stone

Renal stones can be divided into three main types which differ in aetiology and management.

STAGHORN CALCULI

These stones are more common in women and are usually associated with urinary tract infection and renal damage. The major constituent is magnesium ammonium phosphate hexahydrate. Treatment consists of operative removal of the stone and long-term antibiotics to keep the urine sterile postoperatively. This usually means hospital follow-up. If the stone is completely removed and the patient carefully followed up less than five per cent of these stones recur. If however there is incomplete stone removal then the majority of these stones recur very quickly. The long-term morbidity and mortality caused by the continued presence of the stone exceeds that following complete stone removal and urine sterilisation.

RARE METABOLIC STONES

Calcium oxalate

Any case of hypercalcaemia may cause calcium oxalate stone formation. The most important cause to exclude is a para-thyroid adenoma. This occurs in two per cent of patients with stones and five per cent of patients with recurrent stones. The serum calcium taken with the patient fasting, no tourniquet on the arm, and with correction according to the serum proteins is the single most reliable screening test of parathyroid overactivity. The diagnosis is confirmed by the detection of an abnormal concentration of parathormone for the degree of hypercalcaemia, either in venous blood or during selective catheterisation of the neck veins.

Oxalosis

This is a rare inborn error of metabolism. Children with this condition die of renal failure usually by the age of 20.

Uric acid

This has a complex relationship to calcium oxalate calculi (see below). Pure uric acid calculi occur in conditions associated with increased uric acid output, e.g. gout, polycythaemia, lymphoma following cytotoxic drugs. Stone formation can be prevented by long-term therapy with allopurinol 300 mg/day.

Cystine

This is a rare inherited disorder caused by a tubular failure to reabsorb certain amino acids. Cystine stones may present as bilateral renal calculi in children. It is wise to analyse stones from all recurrent stone formers and also to test the urine for cystine. Treatment consists of a high fluid intake and also dietary restriction of foods with a high methionine content, e.g. eggs, milk and meat.

'IDIOPATHIC' CALCIUM OXALATE STONE

Although this stone may occur where there is hypercalcaemia (see above), in most cases no obvious metabolic cause is detectable. Recent work by the Medical Research Council Mineral Metabolism Unit at Leeds suggests that if several urinary crystaloids (e.g. calcium oxalate) and compounds (e.g. glycoaminoglycosans) are examined in isolation no obvious abnormality is found but if the concentration of these compounds is considered together patients with stones are significantly different from controls (Fig. 14.2). The increased incidence of upper urinary tract calculi seen throughout the developed world has also to be explained. The Leeds group have further evidence that these urine constituents are out of balance to a greater degree in patients who have high animal protein food intake. It is interesting to note that as a result of recent inflation in the UK the average annual protein intake has fallen and so has the incidence of stones. Thus the remedy for idiopathic stone formation may lie in health and dietary education rather than any specific therapy. At present, all such patients should be advised to increase their daily fluid intake. This is best done by telling the patient to drink two glasses of fluid with each meal. Vague advice to drink plenty usually does not work.

RECURRENT IDIOPATHIC STONES

In some cases multiple stones are formed but no obvious metabolic abnormality can be detected. It is now becoming clear that many of these are associated with hypercalcuria but without any hypercalcaemia. There appear to be two defects which may result in

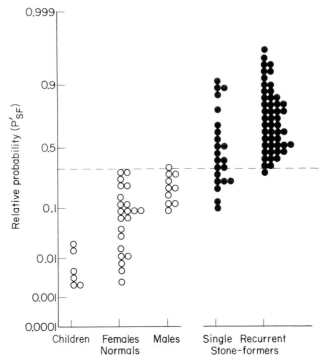

FIG. 14.2   Risk factors in calcium stone disease of the urinary tract. The relative probability of forming stones is calculated by mathematically combining deviations from the mean of the 24-hour urine value of calcium concentration, oxalate concentration, urate concentration, pH, and glycoaminoglycosans. Robertson, W. G. *et al* (1978) Risk factors in calcium stone disease of the urinary tract. *British Journal of Urology*, **50**, 449–454.

this state, the first is hyperabsorption of calcium from the intestine (absorbtive hypercalcuria) and the second is renal leak hypercalcuria. Absorptive hypercalcuria may be distinguished by measuring urinary calcium before and after an oral calcium load and stones may be prevented or reduced in number by cellulose phosphate. Renal leak hypercalcuria may be alleviated by long-term chlorothiazide diuretics. Another group of cases are associated with mild elevations of urinary urate and in these cases calcium oxalate stones may be prevented by long-term allopurinol.

RENAL TUMOUR IN CHILDREN

The developmental renal tumour of children is called a nephroblastoma or Wilm's tumour. Clinical presentation is usually haematuria and an abdominal mass. Treatment is surgical excision of the tumour with radiotherapy and chemotherapy if metastases are present. This multi-modulatory treatment has altered prognosis from an 80 per cent chance of death to an 80 per cent five year survival.

RENAL CELL CARCINOMA IN ADULTS

This is an adenocarcinoma of the kidney. Twenty per cent of cases present with loin pain, haematuria and an abdominal mass. This

TABLE 14.1 Tumour-associated syndromes.

Findings	Per cent of renal tumour patients with this finding	Explanation
Raised ESR	55	Changes in serum proteins associated with many tumours
Hypertension	37	Secretion of renin by tumour
Anaemia	36	Depression of erythropoesis plus or minus haematuria
Weight loss	34	Tumour metabolites depress appetite
Pyrexia	17	Circulating pyrogens
Abnormal liver function	14	This may disappear after nephrectomy
Raised alkaline phosphatase	10·1	Secreted by tumour?
Hypercalcaemia	4·9	Parathormone secretion by tumour
Polycythaemia	3·5	Erythropoietin secretion
Neuromyopathy	3·2	Tumour-associated antibodies to nerve tissue
Amyloidosis	2	Possibly associated with immunological reactions to the tumour

however is a late presentation; approximately 30 per cent of patients present earlier with one of the tumour-associated syndromes (Table 14.1).

Investigations are performed to determine the stage of the tumour and the state of the patient so that rational treatment can be decided.

THE STAGE OF LOCAL INVASION

In order that treatments may be compared the stage of local invasion is ascertained and the tumour given a T category (Fig. 14.3). Venography is usually necessary to exclude invasion of the inferior vena cava.

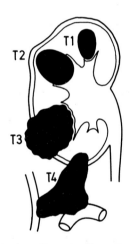

FIG. 14.3   Clinical staging of renal cell carcinoma (T Category). D. M. Wallace, G. D. Chisholm and W. F. Hendry (1975) TNM classification for urological tumours (UICC) 1974, *British Journal of Urology*, **47**, 1–12.

THE STAGE OF LYMPH NODE INVOLVEMENT (N CATEGORY)

This is determined by examination of the mediastinum on the chest X-ray and by abdominal ultrasound (or CAT scan) (Fig. 14.4).

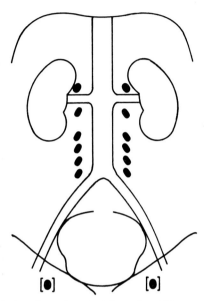

FIG. 14.4 Regional nodes draining the kidney and testis (N category). D. M. Wallace, G. D. Chisholm and W. F. Hendry (1975) TNM classification for urological tumours (UICC) 1974, *British Journal of Urology*, **47**, 1–12.

THE PRESENCE OF METASTASES (M CATEGORY)

A skeletal survey is more sensitive than a bone scan in the detection of bony metastases of renal cell carcinoma. Tumours of the breast, bronchus, kidney, thyroid and prostate all spread to bone. Chest X-ray, often with whole lung tomography, will define pulmonary metastases. Liver function tests and a liver scan may show liver metastases.

THE DEGREE OF MALIGNANCY OF THE TUMOUR

This is usually determined by examination of the operative specimen. In general, anaplastic tumours have a poorer prognosis than better differentiated tumours.

THE GENERAL CONDITION OF THE PATIENT

Radical nephrectomy with radiotherapy and chemotherapy may be appropriate for a 40-year-old man but inappropriate for an 85-year-old man with bronchitis and heart disease. Remember that many solid tumours produce metabolites (Table 14.1) which affect the patient generally. Renal tumours are particularly prone to produce asociated syndromes and most of these syndromes are entirely reversible if the primary tumour is removed before there has been any secondary spread.

The above five considerations apply when planning treatment for any tumour of any organ of the body.

Diagnosis

Diagnosis is made by showing a mass on the kidney on intravenous urography and confirming solidity with an ultrasound. If the ultrasound shows a simple cyst, this can be dealt with by aspiration under ultrasound control. Occasionally, a renal carcinoma is cystic and a mass should only be considered to be benign if it completely disappears following aspiration and if no malignant cells are detected on cytological examination of the aspirate. Arteriography is not usually indicated for diagnosis but it is helpful to embolise the renal artery at arteriography to reduce the tumour size and reduce the operative blood loss.

Treatment

The definitive treatment is surgical excision of the tumour. The five year survival rate for all grades of renal cell carcinoma is approximately 30 per cent. Adjuvant chemotherapy has not yet been properly evaluated; disappointing results have been obtained with the alkylating agents, nitrozoureas, antimetabolite drugs and cisplatinum when used as single agents. As no effective single agents have been found, it is not surprising that multiple agent chemotherapy and adjuvant chemotherapy has also been disappointing.

Attempts have been made to boost the immune response against renal cancer by injecting BCG vaccine or lymphycyte transfer factor and some early results are encouraging but must be confirmed by controlled trials.

There is also some evidence that hormonal therapy may slow the progress of renal cell carcinoma. In a survey of 356 renal carcinoma patients given progesterone-like hormone, eight per cent showed some response. Progesterones are often used because unlike cytotoxic agents, side-effects are minimal; whether such treatment benefits the patient more than the doctor is debatable.

When assessing any treatment for renal carcinoma, it must be borne in mind that spontaneous regression of both the primary tumour and metastases may occur in 0·3 per cent of cases. This is more apt to occur with lung metastases than with bony ones.

OTHER RENAL TUMOURS

1. Transitional cell cancer of the renal pelvis. Transitional cell cancer is dealt with in the section on bladder cancer.
2. Rare tumours
   (a) Adenoma.
   (b) Sarcoma. This tumour arises from the renal connective tissues.
   (c) Angiomyolipoma.
3. Secondary tumours. Blood spread from carcinoma of bronchus and breast may occur as well as lymphatic spread from carcinoma of stomach and pancreas.

POINTS OF EMPHASIS

● Before performing nephrectomy for major renal trauma it is essential to confirm the presence of a healthy contralateral kidney.

● Symptomatic pelviureteric obstruction usually requires surgery. The condition may be bilateral.

● The development of infection in an obstructed kidney is an indication for immediate surgery.

● Staghorn calculi should be treated with complete surgical removal of the stone and postoperative long-term chemotherapy to maintain a sterile urine.

● Five per cent of patients with recurrent stones have hyperparathyroidism.

● Patients with a tendency to stone formation of unknown aetiology should be advised to drink two glasses of fluid with each meal.

● Thirty per cent of patients with renal adenocarcinoma present with a tumour-associated syndrome.

● Rational treatment of renal tumours depends upon the assessment of the patient's general condition, the stage of local invasion, the stage of the lymph node involvement, the presence of metastases and the degree of malignancy of the tumour.

CHAPTER 15

The ureter

INVESTIGATION OF URETERIC ANATOMY

The ureter is usually visualised on the later films of the intravenous urogram series. Peristaltic waves mean that the whole length is rarely seen; if the whole length is seen on one film this may indicate obstruction. If the renal function is too poor to give enough contrast density on the intravenous urogram, the ureter can be visualised in one of three ways.

Antegrade ureteric study. Contrast is injected into the renal pelvis by direct needle puncture. The technique is useful when there is a dilated pelvis.

Retrograde ureterogram. A thin catheter is passed up the ureter through a cystoscope.

Ascending ureterogram. A bulb catheter is placed in the end of the ureter and contrast injected up the ureter.

INVESTIGATION OF URETERIC FUNCTION

Ureteric peristalsis may be viewed using the image intensifier, thus minimising X-ray dosage either during an intravenous urogram series or during a ureterogram. If the ureter is encased in fibrous tissue as in retroperitoneal fibrosis there can be a lack of motility without any dilatation. Ureteric contractions can be measured using a small pressure transducer mounted on a ureteric catheter or by measuring pressure in the renal pelvis at open operation. If reflux of urine up the ureter from the bladder is suspected this can be diagnosed by a micturating cystogram: the bladder is filled with contrast through a urethral catheter. The catheter is removed and the ureters are screened during voiding, the appearance of contrast in the ureter indicating reflux.

MEGAURETER

There are two types of megaureter:
1. Obstructed. In this case there is a failure of conduction of the peristaltic wave in the lower ureter resulting in functional obstruction (comparable with Hirschsprung's disease). This usually presents in (female) children with haematuria, fever and loin pain. Treatment is to restore renal function. If this is severely compromised, it may require the insertion of nephrostomy tubes to drain the kidneys. Once renal function has stabilised the ureters are freed surgically of adhesions and reimplanted.
2. Megaureter associated with vesicoureteric reflux.

VESICOURETERIC REFLUX

Primary reflux is usually diagnosed in children and occurs when there has been a failure of maturation of the normally competent ureterovesical junction. Secondary reflux is associated with obstruction to the outflow of the bladder.

The most important effect of reflux is spread of infection from the bladder to the kidney. Infection is more likely if there is also a bladder outflow problem with associated residual urine. Most of the damage to the kidney from reflux happens within the first five years of life. In order for reflux to result in renal damage it seems probable that there must be associated abnormalities of the renal papillae (page 62). Girls are more often affected than boys. In advanced cases these children may present with renal failure but the usual presentation is with symptoms of cystitis, fever and loin pain. Reflux in adults is less common but may occasionally require treatment because of deteriorating renal function or loin pain.

Most children with reflux can be managed by surgical procedures to ensure free bladder drainage (e.g. treatment of associated urethral valves) and also by measures to prevent urine infections. It is not usually necessary to reimplant the ureters but severe cases may require operation to prevent further reflux. Usually the degree of reflux lessens as the child gets older and this has to be borne in mind before contemplating surgical reimplantation of ureters in children.

URETERIC INJURY

The ureter may occasionally be involved in association with other abdominal injury, e.g. following a road traffic accident. The ureter is at risk during hysterectomy as it crosses the base of the broad ligament. The ureter is also at risk following attempted stone removal by a ureteric basket if the stone is too high. Treatment is immediate surgical repair of the injury.

URETERIC OBSTRUCTION

Within the lumen

The most common cause of obstruction is the passage of a renal stone. This gives the classical symptoms of colicky loin pain radiating to the groin (ureteric colic, Fig. 2.1). Sloughed renal papillae following analgesic abuse or blood clots from a bleeding renal pelvic tumour may also cause colic.

Arising from the ureteric wall

Transitional cell cancer of the urothelial lining of the ureter causes insidious ureteric obstruction not usually associated with ureteric colic but with a dull loin pain of renal distribution. Cases of gradual ureteric obstruction usually present with chronic failure of the affected kidney and dull loin ache because of renal distention.

Any mass which presses on the ureter may cause obstruction. Examples are secondary deposits of para-aortic glands, other masses such as an aortic aneurysm with its associated fibrosis or a cancer from the prostate, bladder or cervix infiltrating the lower end of the ureter.

Retroperitoneal fibrosis

In this strange condition the ureter becomes sheathed with fibrous tissue. The clinical presentation is with renal failure. In approximately half of the cases there is an abdominal malignancy stimulating the fibrosis but in the rest usually no cause can be found. This type of fibrosis is known to occur after use of various drugs. The classical example is methysergide which was once widely used to treat migraine. Treatment is to free the ureter from the fibrosis; the operation is called ureterolysis.

POINTS OF EMPHASIS

● The most important effect of reflux is spread of infection from the bladder to the kidney.

● Most children with ureteric reflux can be managed with long-term antibiotics to keep the urine sterile.

● The ureter is easily injured during hysterectomy; if this happens, treatment is immediate surgical repair.

● The commonest cause of ureteric obstruction is the passage of a renal stone.

CHAPTER 16

The bladder

INVESTIGATION OF ANATOMY

Direct inspection of the bladder and urethra is possible with the cystoscope and urethroscope. In many cases treatment can also be carried out endoscopically, e.g. fulguration of a bladder tumour or litholapaxy (crushing of a bladder stone). The size and shape of the bladder can be visualised on the late film of an intravenous urogram series or by introducing contrast into the bladder via a urethral catheter (cystogram).

INVESTIGATION OF BLADDER FUNCTION

Bladder emptying

The post-voiding film on the intravenous urogram series will sometimes show whether the bladder has been completely emptied. More accurate information is gained by screening the patient during voiding (a micturating cystogram). The residual urine can also be measured by a catheter passed into the bladder immediately after voiding.

Bladder accommodation

The normal bladder is able to accommodate 350 ml of urine without the person being aware of the need to void. When this accommodation fails symptoms of frequency and nocturia may occur. The failure to accommodate a normal volume of urine may be a motor or sensory problem. This failure to accommodate can be

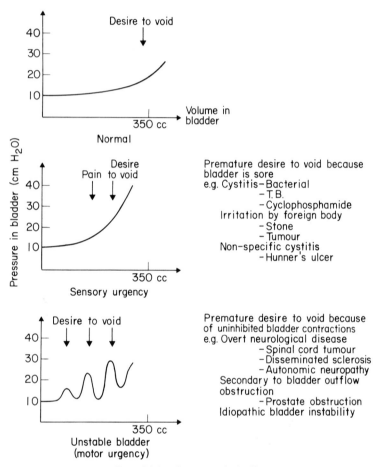

FIG. 16.1 Cystometric findings.

measured by recording pressures within the bladder during bladder filling and emptying (cystometrogram) (Fig. 16.1).

Alterations in bladder function may be accompanied by abnormalities of urethral relaxation. In order to define the problem, cystometry can be done while the bladder is filled and during voiding and at the same time urethral pressure recordings are obtained. This investigation is even further refined by using X-ray contrast as the filling media and screening during voiding with simultaneous pressure, flow and electromyogram measurements.

ALTERATION IN BLADDER FUNCTION

Idiopathic bladder instability

The symptoms of frequency and nocturia reflect bladder overactivity but do not necessarily mean infection. In cases where there is no obvious local bladder irritation and urine is persistently sterile with no pyuria, idiopathic bladder instability should be suspected. This condition is commoner in women than in men. Minor degrees of bladder instability are detectable in approximately ten per cent of women. In severe cases there is typically a history of enuresis often into the teens and subsequently persistent nocturia. The contractions may be so strong as to cause urgency and urge incontinence. Treatment is unsatisfactory as the underlying aetiology is not understood. Some relief is obtained from anticholinergic drugs such as probanthine although side-effects, e.g. dryness of mouth, may be a problem.

Incontinence

Incontinence may occur if the urethral sphincter is too weak or if the bladder has inappropriately powerful contractions, or is over-filled.

URETHRAL SPHINCTER WEAKNESS

This may occur as a consequence of neurological disease, e.g. spinal cord tumour, or may be the result of invasion of the sphincters by tumour. The most common example of this latter situation is carcinoma of the prostate growing downwards into the urethral sphincters. Injury to the urethral sphincter may occur following childbirth or following urethral trauma. Urethral trauma is almost solely confined to men, e.g. urethral rupture following fractured pelvis after a motor cycle accident. The symptoms of sphincter weakness are leakage on stress such as laughing, coughing or changing position. In severe cases there is continuous dribbling incontinence.

POWERFUL BLADDER CONTRACTIONS

It is sometimes very difficult to distinguish this type of incontinence from sphincter weakness incontinence described above. Careful history taking may reveal urgency prior to incontinence. Often the two types of incontinence are mixed. Misdiagnosis of the cause for incontinence is one of the most common reasons for failure of symptomatic improvement following repair operations in women with prolapse. Usually a cystometrogram will distinguish the type of incontinence and this investigation is now increasingly being used in the preoperative evaluation of women prior to repair operations.

OVERFLOW INCONTINENCE

In these cases the bladder is full to capacity with the result that there is continuous dribbling incontinence. The situation is seen if the bladder is paralysed secondary to neurological disease. Temporary bladder paralysis may occur following general anaesthetic and surgery; these cases usually resolve with two or three days of catheter drainage. Chronic urinary retention with overflow incontinence is one of the presenting features of prostatic obstruction. Incomplete bladder emptying increases the liability to urinary infection and bladder stone formation.

ANATOMICAL ABNORMALITIES OF THE BLADDER

Congenital abnormalities are rare. A congenital diverticulum has all layers of the bladder musculature in its wall. Diverticula may be acquired following bladder outflow obstruction; these have no muscle in their walls. Once a diverticulum becomes large, bladder emptying is compromised because instead of the urine passing out through the urethra during a bladder contraction the diverticulum fills instead thereby predisposing to infection. Tumours may occur in acquired diverticula and have a poor prognosis because of their thin walls.

BLADDER TRAUMA

Bladder rupture may occur following a road traffic accident, particularly if the patient has been drinking. Treatment is surgical exploration and repair with drainage through a suprapubic catheter until the bladder has healed.

BLADDER CANCER

The renal pelvis, ureter, bladder and urethra are lined by transitional cell epithelium. Transitional cell cancers may arise anywhere from this epithelium. Those cancers within the bladder have a better prognosis than those elsewhere mainly because they are more accessible to diagnose and treat and also because the bladder wall is thicker.

Incidence

Transitional cell cancer of the bladder is the fifth most common tumour in the UK after cancer of the lung, colo-rectal, breast and stomach. The male–female ratio is 3:1. There appears to have been an increase in incidence in recent years which may be related to environmental factors.

Aetiology

Various chemicals are now known to increase the chances of transitional cell cancer (Table 16.1).

Presenting features

Most cases present with painless haematuria. Widespread bladder tumour irritates the bladder causing symptoms of cystitis which are resistant to antibiotics. Some patients present with loin pain consequent on ureteric obstruction or pain elsewhere because of invasion of neighbouring organs. The patient with advanced disease may be anorexic or cachectic.

Assessment of the tumour

Investigations are tailored to discover the extent of the tumour.

THE STAGE OF LOCAL INVASION

In order to be able to offer rational treatment it is useful to define the stage of local invasion according to the T category (Fig. 16.2).

TABLE 16.1 Chemicals now known to increase the incidence of transitional cell cancer.

Compound	Evidence
Phenacetin	Patients in Sweden with phenacetin nephropathy are now developing transitional cell cancers.
Unknown	The incidence of transitional cell cancer is higher along certain rivers in Yugoslavia. There is also a high incidence of nephropathy in the same areas (Balkan nephropathy). The aetiological agent is unknown.
Bracken fern (*Pteridium aquilum*)	Cattle in Turkey eating the shoots of this fern develop transitional cell cancer of the bladder. Similar cattle elsewhere do not develop this.
Aniline dyes	Men working in factories developed transitional cell cancer of the bladder.
Metabolites of 2-naphthylamine	1. Dogs given this develop transitional cell cancer of the bladder. A portion of dog bladder isolated from the urine does not develop transitional cell cancer even when the dog is fed this compound.
	2. This substance is used as an antioxidant to harden rubber. Men working in chemical, rubber and cable industries were at risk until this substance was banned. Rat catchers, sewage workers and lens grinders also used to handle these compounds and had a high incidence of bladder cancer.
Benzidine	Benzidine was until recently used to test for occult blood in hospitals.
Smoking	Smokers have an increased tendency compared with non-smokers to develop transitional cell cancer of the bladder.

This is done by bimanual examination under anaesthesia and cystoscopy.

LYMPHATIC INVOLVEMENT (N CATEGORY)

This is difficult to define as no accurate techniques exist. Lymphography has a 30 per cent false positive and negative rate compared with the findings from lymph node dissection operations (Fig. 16.3).

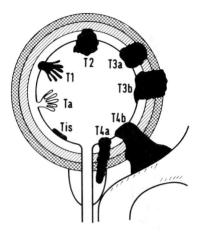

FIG. 16.2 Staging of bladder cancer (T category). This clinical staging is determined by cystoscopic finding and bimanual examination under anaesthetic. G. D. Chisholm *et al* (1980) TNM (1978) in bladder cancer: use and abuse. *British Journal of Urology*, **52**, 500–05.

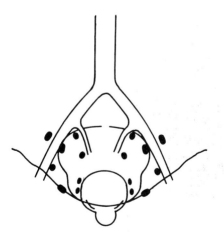

FIG. 16.3 Regional node drainage of bladder and prostate. D. M. Wallace, G. D. Chisholm and W. F. Hendry (1975) TNM classification for urological tumours (UICC) 1974. *British Journal of Urology*, **47**, 1–12.

METASTATIC SPREAD (M CATEGORY)

This is determined by physical examination, chest X-ray, bone scan and liver function tests.

THE DEGREE OF MALIGNANCY OF THE TUMOUR

This is particularly important to define in bladder tumour cases. These tumours often present early with haematuria and some highly malignant tumours are seen at an early stage. The highly anaplastic T2 tumour should be treated in a very different way from the well-differentiated T2 tumour. Thus in the former case there is a likelihood of metastases and consideration is given to adjuvant chemotherapy in addition to local control by endoscopy or radiotherapy; in the latter case endoscopic control is usually successful.

THE GENERAL CONDITION AND AGE OF THE PATIENT

Following failed endoscopic treatment and radiotherapy it may become necessary to remove the bladder (cystectomy) in order to attempt to cure the patient. This type of aggressive surgery is obviously inappropriate in a frail cachectic elderly patient.

Treatment

Sixty per cent of patients with bladder tumours present with localised histologically well-differentiated tumours and are best treated endoscopically. Once the tumour has been diathermied the patient should be observed cystoscopically at intervals for at least ten years because the disease is multifocal and recurs. Observations should also include periodic intravenous urography to demonstrate the upper tract. Every cystoscopy should be accompanied by urethroscopy.

The other 40 per cent of cases have poor grade tumours or advanced tumours on presentation. Treatment is controversial. In general the local bladder lesion is best dealt with by radiotherapy and metastases may be prevented by chemotherapy. Unfortunately despite the many chemotherapeutic agents available few have been properly evaluated. Systemic methotrexate and possibly cisplatinum appear to improve some cases. Widespread superficial tumour in the bladder may respond to local cytotoxic bladder instillations, e.g. epodyl or thiotepa.

In those cases where local treatment fails and there are no metastases or where there are severe local symptoms such as haematuria or incontinence from bladder contracture the treatment of choice is cystectomy. The bladder, urethra and lower one-third of the ureters are removed and the ureters drained to the abdominal skin by an isolated segment of small intestine (ileal conduit). Following cystectomy and ileal loop diversion patients require periodic follow-up with intravenous urography to check the upper tract. A particular complication of cystectomy is reabsorption of acid waste products of urine through the small intestinal wall. This occurs if the patient becomes dehydrated for any reason or if the ileal loop becomes obstructed. Such patients should be encouraged to have a good fluid intake.

Other tumours of the bladder

Squamous cell cancer of the bladder may occur in association with chronic urinary infection, bladder stones, squamous metaplasia of a transitional cell cancer or schistosomiasis. Approximately three per cent of cases of bladder cancer in this country have squamous cell lesions whereas in Egypt, where schistosomiasis is endemic, the majority of lesions are squamous cell. These tumours are difficult to treat because they are usually resistant to radiotherapy and often too advanced for excision.

Occasionally a primary adenocarcinoma of the bladder is seen; these arise either from the trigone or from the urachal remnant.

The bladder may be involved by direct spread in cases of colorectal cancer or cancer of the cervix.

POINTS OF EMPHASIS

● Incontinence may occur if there is urethral sphincter weakness, inappropriate powerful bladder contractions or over-filling of the bladder.

● Instability of the bladder is a common cause of failure of operations for stress incontinence.

● Transitional cell carcinoma of the bladder is the fifth most common cancer in the UK.

● Haematuria is the commonest presenting symptom of bladder carcinoma and should always be investigated quickly in all patients.

● Urinary frequency resistant to antibiotic treatment is the second most common presentation of bladder cancer.

● All cases of transitional cell cancer of the bladder need long-term follow-up because the disease is recurrent and multi-focal.

CHAPTER 17

Diseases of the prostate

PHYSIOLOGY

The prostate gland is situated at the base of the bladder around the urethra. The gland enlarges at puberty under the influence of androgens. The secretions comprise one-fifth of the volume of the ejaculate, the other four-fifths are largely composed of seminal vesicular secretion. Enzymes secreted by the prostate cause the seminal fluid to clot and subsequently liquify. The clot of semen can be gripped by the urethral peristaltic wave allowing forward ejaculation and may also help by sticking the semen to cervical mucus.

INVESTIGATION OF ANATOMY

The prostate can be examined by palpation per rectum. Assessment is made of the size, consistency (soft, firm or hard), and contour (smooth or knobbly). The interior of the prostate can be inspected through the urethroscope. New ultrasound techniques using a rectal ultrasound probe with radial scanning allow a more objective assessment of prostate size and consistency.

PROSTATITIS

This is usually a sequel of previous venereal disease. Such men have chronic perineal discomfort often associated with a slight urethral discharge. On rectal examination the prostate feels boggy and tender and on seminal examination there are many white cells and often, although not always, organisms on culture. Treatment is long-term antibiotics, drugs to relax spasm of the bladder neck (e.g. phenoxybenzamine if the patient's cardiovascular state allows), and prostatic massage. Many men with chronic perineal pain and urgency are labelled as having prostatitis without all of these features. Some of these men have idiopathic bladder neck obstruction. Such cases can be diagnosed by the findings of high intravesical pressure and low flows on cystometry combined with observation of the bladder neck at cystoscopy. In other cases no basis for symptoms can be discovered and psychiatric assessment may become necessary.

BENIGN PROSTATIC HYPERTROPHY

Incidence

There is a ten per cent chance of a Caucasian man needing prostatic surgery if he lives until the age of 80. Some races, notably the Bantu in Africa and the Japanese, appear to have a lower incidence. Most operations are performed between the ages of 60 and 75 but the occasional man develops prostatic obstruction in his 40's.

Clinical features

SYMPTOMS ASSOCIATED WITH URINARY OBSTRUCTION

One of the first symptoms of prostatic enlargement is deterioration in the power of the urine stream. As the disease progresses there may be hesitancy, post-micturition dribbling and spraying of the urine stream. All of these symptoms are the direct consequence of the prostatic enlargement causing narrowing and distortion of the urethra.

SYMPTOMS OF BLADDER INSTABILITY

As the obstruction becomes more severe the bladder develops an unstable response resulting in the additional symptoms of frequency and nocturia (page 261).

SYMPTOMS OF BLADDER FAILURE

In many cases the power of the bladder to overcome the outflow obstruction is insufficient resulting in progressive failure to void completely and a large residual urine (see page 262).

CHRONIC RETENTION WITH OVERFLOW

In this situation the bladder becomes fully distended and there is a constant leakage of urine. Often bladder sensation has become dulled by months of over-distention with large residual urines and such patients may have little discomfort. The ureters are usually dilated with consequent renal failure. Thus the clinical picture is an elderly man, usually dishevelled, covered in uraemic frost, with urine soaked clothes and a large bladder palpable.

ACUTE RETENTION

In these cases there is usually a previous history suggesting prostatic obstruction and a sudden decompensating factor such as an operation (post-anaesthetic muscle atony), overstretching of the bladder because no toilet facilities are available (e.g. long-distance coach journey), or an unusually high fluid load (e.g. after diuretic therapy or alcohol consumption). The bladder distention is painful and it is said that there is no more grateful patient than the one who has an acute retention relieved by catheterisation.

HAEMATURIA

This occurs in about 20 per cent of patients with benign hypertrophy, presumably due to rupture of engorged prostatic veins. It should be remembered that the common condition of benign prostatic hypertrophy may be associated with other common conditions such as transitional cell cancer of the bladder and any attack of haematuria should not be dismissed without investigation.

POTENCY

Approximately 50 per cent of men claim potency at the time of their prostatectomy (see Fig. 19.1). This potency is unaffected by prostatectomy in the vast majority of cases irrespective of the type of operation.

Surgical treatment

There is no medical treatment to shrink the prostate and no preventive treatment. Surgery is best performed as an elective procedure before the development of acute retention or of significant renal failure. The justification for surgery will depend upon such factors as the severity of the symptoms, the presence of renal impairment, the age of the patient and his general medical condition. There are two types of operative approach:

1. Transurethral resection, where the prostate is removed endoscopically. This is more appropriate for medium and small-sized prostates. The mortality from transurethral resection is half of that of open surgery.
2. Open prostatectomy. A suprapubic incision is made and the prostate is enucleated. After both types of prostatectomy the patient requires urethral catheter drainage for two or three days until any haematuria has cleared.

Complications of prostatectomy

Complications after any surgical operation should be considered under two headings.

COMPLICATIONS COMMON TO ANY SURGICAL PROCEDURE

Immediate

Primary haemorrhage can be a problem after transurethral resection if too ambitious a resection is carried out encroaching on the periprostatic veins.

Later

Infection, secondary haemorrhage, pulmonary collapse, chest infection, deep vein thrombosis and pulmonary embolism may all occur after prostatectomy. These complications are reduced by good nursing care including early mobilisation of the patient and postoperative chest physiotherapy.

SPECIAL COMPLICATIONS OF PROSTATECTOMY

The special complication of note is incontinence. This is uncommon if the prostatectomy is carried out by an experienced surgeon; however, for no obvious reason there is a small incidence of incontinence presumably secondary to sphincter damage. Any case of post-prostatectomy incontinence should be evaluated by cystoscopy and by urodynamic tests because in some cases incontinence is caused by continued obstruction either from residual prostate glandular tissue or post-prostatectomy urethral stricture.

CARCINOMA OF THE PROSTATE

Incidence

Approximately 160 men per million of population die each year from carcinoma of the prostate. The incidence figures for this disease are confounded by the fact that post-mortem studies reveal that the majority of men over the age of 80 who die from other causes have latent foci of carcinoma in their prostates. This must be borne in mind when deciding treatment based on an incidentally discovered focus, e.g. a small focus in a prostatectomy sample from a patient operated on for supposed benign hypertrophy.

Clinical features

SYMPTOMS OF PROSTATISM

In many cases the symptoms are indistinguishable from those of benign prostatic hypertrophy (poor stream, hesitancy, post-micturition dribbling, frequency and nocturia). If the tumour is causing obstruction, treatment is by transurethral resection of the obstructing tissue in addition to any treatment designed to control the tumour.

SYMPTOMS FROM LOCAL INVASION

The cancer may grow directly into the urethral sphincters resulting in incontinence. This distressing symptom is very difficult to palliate. Direct spread to involve the lower end of each ureter can result in the patient presenting with uraemia.

SYMPTOMS FROM METASTASES

Prostatic cancer is remarkable because of the tendency towards widespread bony metastases which are usually seen as osteosclerotic areas on X-ray. Patients may present with backache or pain from a pathological fracture. In widespread disease the presenting signs may also be anorexia and cachexia.

Assessment of the tumour

THE STAGE OF LOCAL INVASION (T CATEGORY)

It is perhaps more important to assess the state of local invasion in prostatic cancer than in many other tumours. The reason for this is that the cardiovascular side-effects, including death, may be greater from oestrogens given to control a latent cancer than the mortality and morbidity from the tumour itself if left untreated. Staging is carried out by bimanual examination under general anaesthetic The tumour is given a T category (Fig. 17.1).

LYMPHATIC SPREAD (N CATEGORY)

Occasionally glands may be palpable on physical examination. There is no satisfactory technique for assessing pelvic lymph node spread. Most cases have to be categorised NX, i.e. not possible to assess nodes.

METASTATIC SPREAD (M CATEGORY)

The most accurate way to determine spread to bones is by bone scan and confirmatory X-rays of suspicious areas. Further assessment includes liver function tests, chest X-ray and acid phosphatase estimation. Acid phosphatase is an enzyme secreted by the normal prostate gland but in tumour cases the blood levels are found to be greatly elevated. This tumour marker is a good index of the progress of the disease and is also useful to monitor treatment (Fig. 17.2).

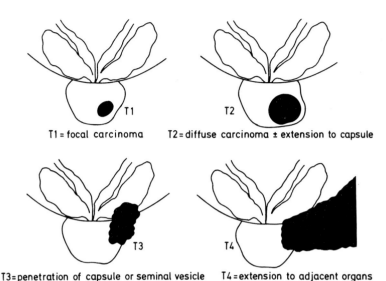

T1 = focal carcinoma   T2 = diffuse carcinoma ± extension to capsule

T3 = penetration of capsule or seminal vesicle   T4 = extension to adjacent organs

FIG. 17.1   Clinical staging of prostatic cancer (T category). This is determined by careful palpation of the prostate, ideally when the patient is under anaesthetic. D. M. Wallace, G. D. Chisholm and W. F. Hendry (1975) TNM classification for urological tumours (UICC) 1974. *British Journal of Urology*, **47**, 1–12.

THE DEGREE OF MALIGNANCY

The degree of malignancy is particularly difficult to assess in prostatic cancer. Well-differentiated tumours tend to have a marked glandular pattern whereas this is lost in poorly differentiated lesions: however, the same tumour may contain areas of differing degrees of malignancy. As a general principle with any cancer the prognosis depends on the area of poorest differentiation.

THE GENERAL CONDITION OF THE PATIENT

A poor general condition is seen either when there is widespread metastatic disease or when there is uraemia consequent on ureteric obstruction or when there is severe coexisting disease.

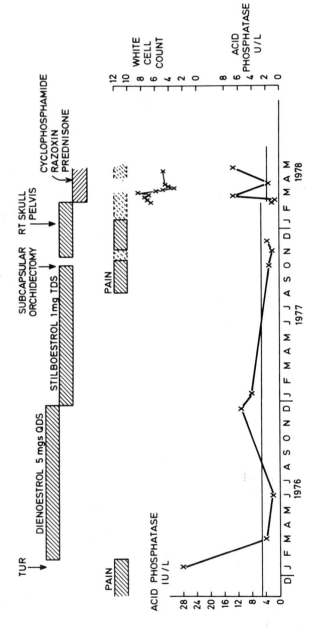

FIG. 17.2 Illustrative case of prostatic cancer showing the use of acid phosphatase as a tumour marker. In this case disease progressed in spite of several types of treatment. A new assay for acid phosphatase (1978) explains the change of scale.

Treatment of prostatic cancer

This depends on the tumour assessment described above.

EARLY LOCALISED DISEASE

In view of the high incidence of asymptomatic localised disease in patients dying of other causes there is considerable doubt as to the best management of these cases. Some will defer treatment until symptoms appear or progression is documented; other surgeons immediately start treatment. Evidence suggests early low dose oestrogen treatment does not alter the ultimate survival but may delay the onset of metastases. Early high dose oestrogen is associated with a greater death rate from complications than from the cancer itself. The place of radiotherapy for early localised disease has yet to be fully evaluated.

LOCALLY ADVANCED DISEASE

Once the cancer has spread locally to invade the periprostatic area, urethral sphincters or base of the bladder, treatment is necessary to relieve symptoms. In the absence of metastases it is probably logical to give radiotherapy although many surgeons will prescribe oestrogens.

METASTATIC DISEASE

Prostatic cancer is under the influence of androgens and first line treatment is either to antagonise androgen production with oestrogen therapy or to deprive the tumour of androgen by subcapsular orchidectomy. The latter treatment has the advantage that there are no feminising side effects and no dangerous cardiovascular side-effects. The subjective response in terms of bone pain is often dramatic and there may be objective response as measured by bone scan. In the event of failure of primary treatment it is reasonable to try chemotherapy although not many agents have been properly evaluated. Hypophysectomy sometimes results in dramatic pain relief after all other therapies have failed.

In addition to the above systemic therapies it may become necessary to treat individual painful bony metastases with radiotherapy.

POINTS OF EMPHASIS

● Prostatic hypertrophy may present as acute or chronic urinary retention.

● The mortality from transurethral prostatectomy is half that of open prostatectomy.

● Symptoms of carcinoma of the prostate and benign prostatic hypertrophy are often indistinguishable.

● Prostatic carcinoma may metastasise widely to bone and on X-ray these are seen as sclerotic deposits.

● Carcinoma of the prostate is a common, incidental finding at post-mortem examination of elderly men who die from other diseases.

● The cardiovascular risks of high dose oestrogens given for localised prostatic cancer outweigh any benefit of therapy.

CHAPTER 18

Diseases of the urethra

ANATOMICAL AND PHYSIOLOGICAL INVESTIGATION

The urethra can be inspected by urethroscopy. This should be done as a routine part of any cystoscopic examination of the bladder and is particularly important in patients with bladder tumours, of whom five per cent have urethral involvement. Sometimes it is not possible to pass a cystoscope because of the stricture, in which case the anatomy can be determined by ascending and descending urethrograms. An ascending urethrogram is an X-ray that is taken while contrast is injected up the urethra and a descending urethrogram is taken when the patient voids the contrast. The function of the urethra can be investigated by a flow rate (this of course reflects bladder power as well as urethral resistance) and also by a urethral pressure profile. Urethral pressure profile is an investigation whereby the pressure within the lumen of the urethra at various points is recorded. This investigation is particularly useful in spinal injury cases where a spastic pelvic floor may result in a very high urethral resistance; such cases can be treated by incision of the spastic sphincter. Postoperative urethral pressure profiles can be done to check that surgery has been successful.

URETHRAL INFLAMMATION

Acute urethritis with penile discharge and dysuria are symptoms usually associated with gonorrhoea. Non-specific urethritis may also cause these symptoms to a lesser degree. These diagnoses should be borne in mind when young patients are attending a urological clinic complaining of dysuria particularly in view of the prevalence of venereal disease (Fig. 18.1). Urethritis also occurs after the passage of a catheter, cystoscope, foreign body or stone.

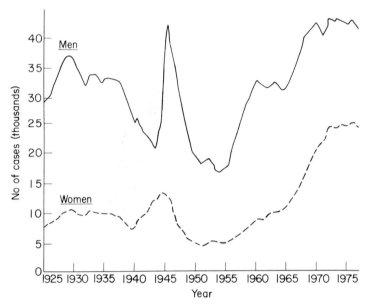

FIG. 18.1 UK prevalence of gonorrhoea. *British Medical Journal* (1979) Sexually transmitted disease surveillance 1978. **2**, 1375.

URETHRAL INJURY

It is rare for women to suffer urethral injury following trauma. Prolapse, particularly after multiple childbirth, may result in urethral distortion with occasional incontinence or urethral discomfort as sequelae.The male urethra is more easily damaged because it is longer and fixed. The two main injuries are:

1. Rupture of the urethra at the apex of the prostate.
2. Rupture of the penile bulba urethra.

Rupture of the urethra at the apex of the prostate

This is usually associated with major injury such as a fracture of the pelvis following a motor-cycle injury. The prostate and bladder are dislocated upwards and there may be extravasation of urine into the periprostatic space. The diagnosis should be suspected in cases of fracture of the pelvis in association with blood at the external penile meatus. Management depends on whether the injury is isolated or part of multiple trauma. In cases of multiple injury the first priority is to replace blood volume and secure an airway. Catheterisation will usually be required in order to manage the patient's fluid balance but there is a real risk of converting a partial urethral tear into a complete rupture, thus when catheterisation becomes necessary this should be done by an experienced surgeon, preferably the urological consultant. If catheterisation is unsuccessful, then exploration in theatre will be required. When the patient is too ill for a full exploration or else there is no experienced surgeon available, the safe initial procedure is suprapubic drainage of the bladder. If experienced help is available, it is better to operate in cases of complete rupture to align the urethra and approximate the ends. Alignment is achieved by passing a urethral catheter and approximation is achieved by a tension suture through the prostate. The decision as to whether the rupture is complete and therefore needing the above repair, or partial and therefore requiring suprapubic drainage only is made by urethroscopy carried out immediately before the incision is made.

In cases where the injury is isolated it is usually safe to observe. If the patient voids the urethra is intact; if the urethra is ruptured, contrary to popular belief, the usual result is retention. If retention occurs, this is managed by urethroscopy and either surgical repair or suprapubic catheterisation as described above.

Many cases of urethral injury develop post-operative urethral stricture which, if long, may require urethroplasty.

Rupture of the penile bulba urethra

This is a less severe injury usually following a fall astride. The rupture may be complete or incomplete. The perineum is bruised and if the patient voids urine it is extravasated into the scrotum rising up the anterior abdominal wall under the deep fascia.

Treatment is by suprapubic catheter drainage and urethrogram to assess the extent of the rupture. If there is a partial rupture the urethra is best left alone as attempts at catheterisation are likely to convert this partial rupture into a complete rupture.

Urethral stricture

Stricture may follow inflammation or trauma. In general short traumatic strictures are much easier to treat than a long inflammatory one. The first step in management is to assess the length of the stricture using urethrograms and urethroscopy. If the stricture is short the best treatment is incision under direct vision using the urethroscopy and urethrotomy knife. Longer strictures may require excision of the diseased segment and end-to-end anastomosis; this is not always possible and some strictures have to be managed by repeated outpatient dilatation using urethral dilators.

CHAPTER 19

Diseases of the penis

DISORDERS OF THE FORESKIN

Phimosis

In this condition there is scarring of the foreskin so that it cannot be retracted fully to reveal the glans penis. This condition may occasionally be so severe as to cause retention of urine. In most cases the only complication is an increased liability to infection beneath the foreskin with subsequent scarring of the glans. These infections tend to cause more trouble with increasing age.

Treatment is by circumcision.

Paraphimosis

If there is a degree of phimosis and the foreskin is retracted (usually during intercourse) the glans may swell up making replacement of the foreskin impossible. This common condition is treated by reduction of the paraphimosis and later circumcision. Reduction of the paraphimosis is achieved by compressing the glans of the penis to reduce the oedema while the patient is under general anaesthetic.

Balanitis

This infection is beneath the foreskin of the glans penis and is often associated with phimosis or with poor personal hygiene.

PROBLEMS WITH ERECTION

Impotence

Impotence occurs with increasing frequency over the age of 40 affecting about 50 per cent of men in their late sixties (Fig. 19.1). In most cases no organic explanation can be found and the younger man may require psychiatric evaluation. Measurement of serum

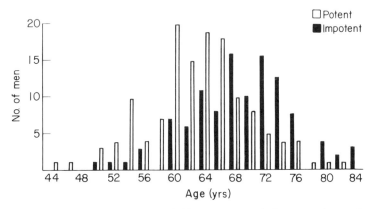

FIG. 19.1 Two hundred and fifty-two men, their age and sexual potency. From Hargreave, T. B and Stephenson, T. P. (1977) Potency and prostatectomy. *British Journal of Urology*, **49**, 683–688.

hormones is unrewarding and non-specific hormone therapy unhelpful. It should be remembered that serious systemic disease may present as impotence or that there may be a specific neurological problem, e.g. autonomic blockage caused by antihypertensive drugs or a diabetic autonomic neuropathy (Table 19.1).

Peyronie's disease

This bizarre disease is a collagen disorder similar to and associated with Dupuytren's contracture of the hand. Plaques of fibrous tissue develop adjacent to the corpora causing bending of the penis during erection. The deformity may render sexual intercourse impossible. Medical treatment is unsatisfactory; in severe cases plastic surgical operations are often successful.

TABLE 19.1   Some causes of impotence.

Psychological	Injury or tumour particularly if temporal lobe involved
CNS	Drugs which depress CNS: barbiturates, alcohol
Spinal cord	Injury or tumour affecting S2–3
Peripheral nerves	Abdomino-perineal resection
S2–3 root	Drug blockage: ganglion blockers
Autonomic nerves	Antihypertensives: Guanethidine, bethanidine, methyldopa, clonidine and some beta adrenoceptor blocking agents
Blood supply	Severe aorto iliac arteriosclerosis Bilateral lumbar sympathectomy
Inappropriate hormones	Lack of androgen: Orchidectomy Excess oestrogen: treatment for carcinoma of prostate

Hypospadias

This is a congenital deformity of the penis where the external urethral meatus opens on the ventral surface. In severe cases the scrotum may be pitted. It is not always appreciated that this deformity is associated with fibrosis on the dorsal aspect of the penis so that during erection the penis is angulated to such an extent as to make intercourse impossible. Treatment is by plastic surgical operation, (1) to bring the urethra to the end of the penis and (2) to correct any penile angulation.

Epispadias

This is a much rarer deformity where the urethra opens on to the dorsal aspect of the penis. In severe cases the whole bladder opens on to the anterior abdominal wall (ectopia vesicae). There is usually an associated failure of symphysis of the pubis. Treatment of severe cases is by plastic surgery shortly after birth; in such cases it is usually necessary to perform a urinary diversion.

CARCINOMA OF THE PENIS

This tumour is a squamous cell cancer usually arising from the glans penis. In most cases the tumour arises under the foreskin in an uncircumcised man. Prognosis depends on the grade of tumour and stage of spread. If the tumour is localised the most effective treatment is by radiotherapy using special moulds to give the required dose to the tumour. Such treatment is followed by as good a cure rate as surgical excision but without having to submit the patient to penile amputation. Penile amputation may be necessary should radiotherapy fail or if there is a massive fungating local tumour. If there is spread to inguinal glands these can also be excised but prognosis is much poorer as secondary squamous cancer is in general resistant to radiotherapy and chemotherapy. It is surprising how many of these patients will ignore their tumour until it is hopelessly advanced; a rather similar situation is seen with reserved old ladies who will deny a very advanced carcinoma of the breast.

CHAPTER 20

Diseases of the testis

MALDESCENT OF THE TESTIS

The testis arises from the urogenital ridge just below the developing kidney and descends shortly before birth to lie in the scrotum. This descent is under the influence of fetal androgens secreted by the developing testes in response to placental gonadotrophins. If the testis is not in the scrotum by one year of age it is unlikely to descend spontaneously. As the child grows older cremasteric muscles develop so that by the age of six there is an apparently higher incidence of undescent because of retractile organs. If the testes do not descend properly there is a higher than normal chance of subsequent malignancy and also infertility. These risks are reduced if orchidopexy is carried out before puberty and very much reduced if orchidopexy is carried out before the age of six years. The inguinal canal and if necessary the abdominal cavity is explored and after the testis has been located it is mobilised sufficiently to allow it to be placed in the scrotum. It is usually necessary to fix the testis in the scrotum to prevent subsequent retraction. There are various types of orchidopexy all of which achieve these objectives. The adult with unilateral high undescent is best advised to have an orchidectomy because of the risk of malignancy and also because that testis will not be contributing towards spermatogenesis. It is often of help to such patients to place a Silastic testicular prosthesis in the scrotum at the time of orchidectomy.

SCROTAL SWELLINGS

It is important to distinguish the various scrotal swellings. An

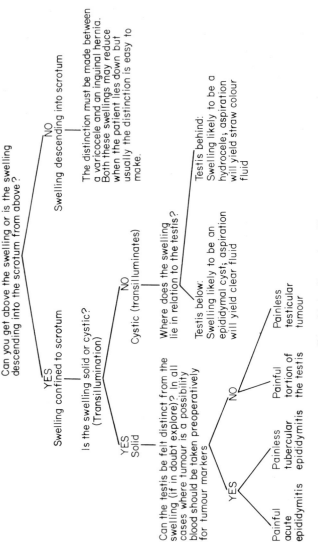

FIG. 20.1   Scrotal swellings.

approach to this is illustrated (Fig. 20.1); it should be remembered that it rarely causes any harm to explore the scrotum surgically for a benign condition but to miss a malignant one can spell disaster for the patient.

EPIDIDYMO-ORCHITIS

Usually the epididymis only is involved becoming acutely painful and distended following some other provoking cause such as a urinary infection. Thus this problem is one of the postoperative complications following prostatic surgery, particularly if the urine becomes infected. There are other much rarer forms of granulomatous orchitis predominantly affecting the testis; these are of unknown aetiology. Painless craggy swelling of the epididymis should suggest the possibility of tuberculosis.

TORSION OF THE TESTICLE

This usually occurs in pubertal boys or young men. Often the testes have a predisposition to tort because of an abnormal horizontal lie. Torsion usually occurs at night and starts with a sudden painful swelling of the testes. It is sometimes difficult to distinguish cases from acute epididymo-orchitis. It is wise if there is any doubt to explore the scrotum. Irreversible testicular damage will occur if testicular torsion is not corrected within six hours whereas it rarely causes any harm to surgically explore an epididymo-orchitis. Treatment is to untwist the testicle surgically and fix both testes to prevent further torsion; both sides should be fixed because the opposite testis usually has the same liability to tort.

TESTICULAR TUMOURS

Testicular tumours arising from the germinal epithelium

Seminomas and teratomas may occur alone or in combination; approximately one patient in seven has a combined tumour. There has been in recent years, an overall increase in the incidence of testicular tumours in the UK, before 1963, 2·3 per hundred thousand men, 1963–1966, 2·74 per hundred thousand, 1966–1971, 3·76 per hundred thousand. The reason for this increase is not known. Testicular tumours are uncommon in non-white races. Previous testicular undescent increases the risk of malignancy 30 times; this risk is substantially reduced if orchidopexy is carried out before the age of six.

TERATOMAS

Teratomas are thought to arise from toti-potential germ cells and may develop into extra-embryonic tumours (choriocarcinoma or yolk sac carcinoma) or intra-embryonic tumour (teratoma). These tumours mainly occur between the ages of 20–30 years. Teratomas in children tend to be well-differentiated and have a benign course.

SEMINOMAS

Seminomas are thought to arise from the germ cells after they are differentiated into spermatogonia. These tumours mainly occur between the ages of 30 and 40.

CLINICAL FEATURES OF TESTICULAR TUMOURS

Most cases present because of testicular swelling. Not infrequently there is a misleading history of minor trauma which is thought by the patient to account for the tumour. Some cases present with advanced secondary spread; the rapid growth of pulmonary metastases in a young man may simulate a pneumonia.

ASSESSMENT OF THE TESTICULAR TUMOURS

Stage of spread

Local invasion up the inguinal cord is uncommon and in most cases the tumour is within the testes or has disseminated widely. The commonly used staging system in the UK is:

Stage 1. Tumour confined to testis.
Stage 2. Abdominal glands (positive lymphangiogram but no other evidence of spread.
Stage 3. Supradiaphragmatic lymphatic spread, e.g. mediastinal mass on chest X-ray or enlarged supraclavicular glands.

Stage 4. Extra-lymphatic spread, e.g. secondaries in lungs, liver or brain.

The degree of malignancy

The most malignant area of the tumour determines prognosis. A teratoma may have several cell lines, some highly anaplastic, and some tending towards differentiation; this accounts for the variegated appearance of these tumours.

The state of the patient

These tumours usually occur in young men with no other illness. It is often reasonable to try heroic treatments to try to save the patient.

Tumour markers

These are particularly important in the diagnosis and management of testicular tumours. Tumour markers are by definition circulating compounds secreted by a tumour or made by the body in response to a tumour. These compounds are present in excessive amounts. Some are recognisable hormones with biological action but many hundreds of compounds are thought to be tumour markers and in most no biological action has been discovered. The important tumour markers in cases of testicular tumour are alpha feto-protein, human chorionic gonadotrophin and lactic dehydrogenase. Blood should be taken for assay of these markers before any surgery to remove a scrotal mass that could be a tumour. If the markers are positive, disappearance after operation is usually a good indication that the tumour has been totally removed. Reappearance of markers during follow-up will often precede overt appearance of metastases and is an indication for treatment. One warning is that these markers may be secreted by one cell line of a multi-cell line teratoma. Disappearance of markers does not always mean that all the tumour has been cleared.

TREATMENT

The primary treatment is to remove the testicular tumour by operation using an inguinal approach and ligating the cord at the internal inguinal ring. In America many surgeons also perform retroperitoneal lymph node dissection but this practice is now decreasing following the discovery of effective chemotherapy. Metastases from seminoma are particularly radiosensitive. The overall three year survival for seminoma is 88 per cent with a 53 per cent three year survival even in the presence of metastases. The treatment of choice for teratoma is now chemotherapy. The new platinum chemotherapeutic agents have increased survival expectancy from the old overall survival figure of 47 per cent at three years (three per cent at three years with metastases) to a similar rate observed for seminoma cases.

Other testicular tumours

Lymphomas may present either as primary or secondary tumours of the testis usually in men over the age of 50. Rare tumours may also arise from Sertoli cells and from interstitial cells. Sometimes these have hormonal effects. A relatively common benign tumour of Mullerian duct origin may arise in the epididymis—the adenomatoid tumour.

INFERTILITY

Until recently it has been common practice to investigate one or other partner of an infertile marriage in isolation. It is now realised that in one-third of couples there are problems in both partners. It is worthwhile noting the minimum requirements of female investigation which are tests (1) to determine whether there is regular ovulation and (2) to prove that the Fallopian tubes are patent.

A man is often judged fertile or not depending on semen analysis; in general, this is unwise because there is no good technique to predict which sperm are fertile.

Types of male infertility

AZOOSPERMIA SECONDARY TO TESTICULAR DAMAGE

In this situation the ejaculate contains no sperm because both testicles have suffered severe damage. This may be secondary to a chromosomal disorder such as Klinefelter's syndrome (XXY) or may be the result of undescended testes or some other non-specific injury. There is no treatment known to restore fertility.

AZOOSPERMIA SECONDARY TO VAS OBSTRUCTION

Obstruction of the vas deferens may be congenital or acquired. Operations to bypass congenital obstruction have a low success rate whereas reversal of vasectomy if done within two years of the original operation carries an 80 per cent chance of success.

OLIGOZOOSPERMIA

Approximately 20 per cent of men attending an infertility clinic are found to have very poor parameters on seminal analysis and testicular biopsy will show that this is secondary to damage to the germinal epithelium. This can occur as a result of testicular undescent, some virus infections including mumps after puberty and also after exposure to certain pesticides but in most cases there is no obvious aetiology. There is no proven effective therapy despite the claim that many hormone treatments are effective. The placebo effect of these treatments should not however be underestimated.

VARICOCELE

Varicose veins may occur in the scrotum above the testis, usually on the left, secondary to a failure of a valve in the testicular vein. Large varicosities associated with a free reflux of blood impair fertility but the precise mechanism for this is not understood. Such cases can be helped by varicocele ligation. Small varicosities not associated with reflux of blood probably do not affect fertility.

EJACULATION PROBLEMS

These have been dealt with in Chapter 10.

ANTISPERM ANTIBODIES

About five per cent of men attending an infertility clinic appear to have circulating antisperm antibodies which may be reduced by steroid therapy. The exact significance of these has not been elucidated but it has been shown that the presence of these antibodies cannot be predicted by routine semen analysis.

POINTS OF EMPHASIS

● The increased instance of infertility and malignancy in an undescended testis can be reduced by orchidopexy, especially if performed under the age of six.

● Orchidectomy is advisable in an adult with a unilateral undescended testis because of the risk of malignancy.

● Where there is doubt, it is advisable to surgically explore solid swellings confined to the scrotum.

● Irreversible damage will occur if testicular torsion is not corrected within six hours whereas little harm results from surgical exploration of a case of epididymo-orchitis.

● Most testicular tumours present before the age of 40.

● Postoperative disappearance of tumour markers suggests, but does not confirm, total tumour resection; reappearance of a marker is an indication for further therapy.

● Metastases from a seminoma are highly radio-sensitive.

● Combination chemotherapy is now the treatment of choice for testicular teratoma.

Subject Index

295